THE PLANTAR FASCIITIS PLAN

Praise from Doctors

"Plantar fasciitis can be a 'real pain' for both patients and medical professionals. This book does a great job of helping both patients and medical professionals not only understand plantar fasciitis but also manage both acute and chronic cases. Dr. Colin Dombroski has done a great job with debunking myths and structuring the book into an easy-to-use tool. I would definitely recommend it."
— DR. TATIANA JEVREMOVIC, MD, CCFP(EM), DIP SPORT
 MED SPORT AND EXERCISE MEDICINE PHYSICIAN

"I have referred innumerable difficult-to-treat patients to Colin with lasting success. This book reinforces why I continue to do so. His stepwise and measured approach is easy to understand and based on solid principles. A great resource."
— DR. FRANK SHIN, MD, CCFP, DIP SPORT MED SPORT AND
 EXERCISE MEDICINE PHYSICIAN

Praise from Patients

"I am pain free because of Colin's wisdom. Buy this book and get your life back."
— LOUISE KARCH, MED, AMC, CMP
 AUTHOR, INTERNATIONAL EDUCATOR, ACCREDITED
 MASTER COACH, AWARD-WINNING CONSULTANT

"Dr. Colin Dombroski is passionate and a professional in his field of helping people recover from plantar fasciitis. His book is easy to read and apply to your life to regain your health and enjoy the activities you love to do."
— BRENDA DE PAUW, BA

"Over the years, I have had a number of sports injuries that have been treated with surgery or physiotherapy. These injuries were painful when they occurred; however, the pain did not continue as with plantar fasciitis. Colin was recommended to me by an orthopedic surgeon for treatment and care of my plantar fasciitis, which I had endured for many months. The explanation of the injury mechanics, the treatment plan, and the orthotics were the solution to a very painful problem. I found Colin to be very knowledgeable, insightful, and personable. I would highly recommend Colin for anyone experiencing foot problems of any nature."
— THEODORE J. MADISON BA, LLB

"I really enjoyed reading your information on plantar fasciitis. It's a great reminder that plantar fasciitis can return (I've already had it twice). I especially liked the pictures of the foot exercises and the reminders that foot exercises are so important. I remain pain free. Thank you, Colin."
— SUSAN McMURRAY

"Colin focuses on the problem and the specific 'pain' points that many of us go through. This drew me in to hear more about what I can do to solve it. The book was very easy to read and follow, and the exercises are easy to understand and to do. I'd recommend *The Plantar Fasciitis Plan* to anyone suffering heel pain."
— NICK DiNARDO

"As an avid golfer and runner of half marathons, when a return bout of plantar fasciitis occurred, I was sidelined from enjoying both these sports. I was referred to Colin and was informed straight up that it would take some time to heal my painful situation, but with proper exercise and custom orthotics, Colin was confident he would get me back to golf and running. He was right! It took about eight months, but I am now back to walking eighteen holes of golf (four to five times per week) and currently in the early stages of getting back into running. I am now pain free from plantar fasciitis and I cannot thank Colin enough for his advise and expertise."

— ROBERT NEILL

"After several consultations with Colin, here is the program that works for me.

1. I always wear shoes/boots that are properly fitted for my feet. I have indoor shoes, outdoor shoes, and winter boots. I have three pairs of orthotics: one for my indoor shoes, one for my outdoor shoes, and one for my winter boots. I never walk anywhere in my bare feet.
2. Colin has recommended many exercises, which I have tried. At the end of the day, I have picked two that I will do because I have time, and they have worked successfully for me. The arch stretch for one minute on each foot is the first one, and then I do the foot massage using my knuckles instead of a tennis ball. I do these two procedures twice a day. Once when I first get out of bed in the morning and once latter in the day after I have been sitting for quite a while. Some of the other exercises were bothering my feet. As Colin says, if it hurts, don't do it.

Bottom line, by wearing proper fitting shoes, having the right orthotics for each shoe, always wearing shoes (don't go barefoot), and doing the above exercises twice a day I have been able to manage my plantar fasciitis successfully with no pain. I only wish I had met Colin sooner, and I certainly have recommended him to other plantar fasciitis suffers."

— JIM COOK

"Plantar fasciitis has really limited my ability to function effectively in sport and slowed down my everyday walking activities due to heel pain. This particular book does an incredible job of being equally accessible to all audiences in terms of breaking down the fundamental understanding of plantar fasciitis. Whether its acute or chronic, minor or severe pain, the chapters really break down the process of getting you back to having "happy feet." In all honesty, if you have been diagnosed with even acute plantar fasciitis, you should get this book. Take the preventative approach and educate yourself before you regret it, because it can be a very long and depressive road to recovery. Colin's book will ensure that you have the wisdom needed to do so."

— RICK MELO
GENERAL MANAGER, LA FITNESS INTERNATIONAL

"The pain I experienced from plantar fasciitis restricted me from the thing I enjoy most in life: playing with my dog. I was unable to walk or run without intense pain. Colin's book was insightful and helped me understand the why and how so I could help myself. I cannot thank Colin and his team enough for giving me back my mobility. Bridget and I both thank you!"

— CHRISTINE ROWE

THE PLANTAR FASCIITIS PLAN

FREE YOUR FEET FROM MORNING PAIN

Get The Best Exercises, Footwear, Orthotic Advice & More to
FEEL BETTER TOMORROW MORNING

COLIN DOMBROSKI

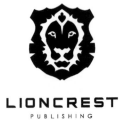

THE PLANTAR FASCIITIS PLAN
Free Your Feet From Morning Pain

ISBN   978-1-61961-518-2   *Paperback*
       978-1-61961-519-9   *Ebook*

INTERIOR DESIGN BY
www.DominiDragoone.com

*To my amazing wife, Cynthia; my fussy-face Lander; and the girls,
thank you for the encouragement and understanding of the countless
hours spent on this project. You are my inspiration.*

*To my parents, thank you will never be enough.
You taught me how to get back up.*

I love you all so very much.

CONTENTS

FOREWORD

A long with death and taxes, the one thing we can all count on is suffering with sore feet at some stage in our lives. Whether you are an elite athlete, a weekend warrior, or a factory worker, foot pain can have a major impact on your performance and quality of life. Plantar fasciitis is arguably the most common cause of foot pain that is best managed through nonoperative modalities. Dr. Colin Dombroski has put together this all-encompassing manual to assist patients and caregivers alike as they work through the diagnosis and management of this frustrating ailment. Knowledge is power and Dombroski certainly empowers his reader with detailed chapters covering the anatomy of the plantar fascia, signs and symptoms of fasciitis, causes, prevention, and leading-edge treatment. Dombroski presents chapter after chapter of highly practical suggestions including the REST protocol, shoe selection, exercises, and workplace prevention strategies. In chapter 13, we are presented the "quick start guide to custom orthotics," which is a fantastic overview that helps the reader make informed decisions. This book is a must read for anyone suffering through plantar fasciitis or hoping to avoid it!

— Dr. Robert Litchfield, MD, FRCSC
Orthopedic Surgeon and Medical Director,
Fowler Kennedy Clinic

DISCLAIMER

This book is intended to supply general educational information only. This book is not intended to be used as a substitute for any kind of professional medical advice. Each patient is unique, and solutions and their results vary. Users should not rely on anything in this book without seeking professional advice from a qualified physician or foot specialist.

Mention of specific companies, organizations, or authorities in this book does not imply endorsement by the author or publisher, nor does mention of specific companies, organizations, or authorities imply that those entities endorse this book, its author, or the publisher.

Any third-party sites that are linked to this book are not under the author's control. The author is not responsible for anything on the linked sites, including—without limitation—any content, links to other sites, any changes to those sites, or any policies those sites may have. The author provides links as a convenience only, and such links do not imply endorsement by the author or publisher, nor does mention of specific companies, organizations, or authorities imply that those entities endorse this book, its author, or the publisher.

MY PLEDGE

Thank you so much for buying *The Plantar Fasciitis Plan: Free Your Feet from Morning Pain.*

Because you've made the choice to help yourself, I'm making a pledge to help those in need. For years, I've been part of a wonderful organization called Operation Walk. The purpose of Op Walk is to provide total joint replacement surgery for people in developing countries. These patients otherwise have little access to care for debilitating bone and joint diseases. For more information, check out operationwalk.ca or my website, **www.thepfplan.com**, where you can see videos of me in action in Ecuador!

Your purchase will buy a pair of shoes for someone in Guatemala or Ecuador. By buying this book, you're now part of a team that helps people unable to walk get back on their feet.

Now let's get you back on yours.

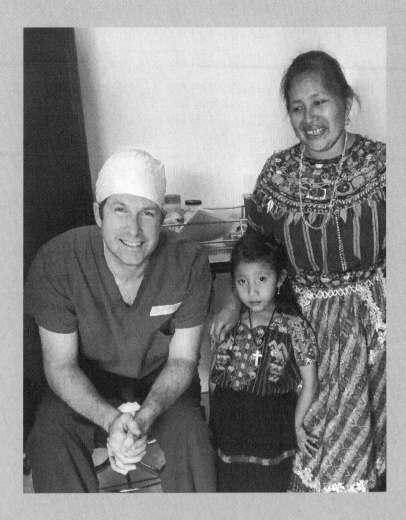

OPERATION WALK
www.operationwalk.ca
www.thepfplan.com

THE PLANTAR FASCIITIS PLAN

INTRODUCTION

Do any of these sound like you?

"I have pain in my heel when I get up first thing in the morning."

"My first ten steps really hurt."

"I can be active as much as I want to be, but afterward, I'm crawling in pain just to be able to get to the bathroom."

"I've been told to stop all of my activity because I'm sore and now I've gained twenty pounds. "

"I have a hard time going to work. I can barely get through my shift."

"My heel hurts so much, I have a hard time concentrating."

If any of these complaints sound like you, you almost certainly have plantar fasciitis—pain in the heel of the foot. I hate to hear my patients tell me they're in ongoing pain, because I know they don't have to be. That's why I wrote this book.

Plantar fasciitis (fash-eee-EYE-tiss), or PF for short, is a common foot problem—one that's easily managed in its early stages. Sadly, by the time a patient comes to me, the problem usually hasn't been managed as well as it could have been. My job is to help patients with recent or long-standing cases of PF recover. I've been a clinical specialist, a Canadian-certified pedorthist, for over twelve years. About 60 percent of my day is spent dealing with patients who have plantar fasciitis. Over the course of my career, I've treated some five thousand cases of plantar fasciitis, successfully for the vast majority. The earlier we intervene, the more likely you are to get better. I've been able to help even people who did everything right but still didn't get better.

There's no one way to get plantar fasciitis, and there's no one definitive way to treat it. But don't despair. In my experience, only about 3 to 5 percent of cases remain chronic over time. With good individualized treatment, 95 percent of my patients will get better. The only real question is how long it will take. Some people only need to see me once. I give them some basic home-based therapy things to do and in six weeks they'll be back at 100 percent function, with no pain. Other people will take longer. I've had some patients who have seen four or five different specialists, spent thousands of dollars over several years, and are actually worse off than when their symptoms first started. Even these patients can almost always be helped.

HOW YOU CAN FEEL BETTER TOMORROW MORNING

The hallmark of plantar fasciitis is pain after rest. You get up in the morning, and your first ten or twenty steps feel like someone's taking an ice pick and shoving it into the bottom of your heel. Some people say that it's a mild ache. Other people literally have to crawl to the bathroom in the morning. But once you've taken those first steps, your foot feels better. Why? Those first steps hurt so much because you're reinjuring your foot after overnight rest. Those steps are when you're doing most of the damage for the rest of the day. What I'm going to give you in this book are strategies to reduce your morning pain and keep it from coming back. Some people get atypical plantar fasciitis, where the pain is felt more toward the end of the day. The strategies in this book work regardless of the time of day you feel the pain.

The information about plantar fasciitis on the Internet and elsewhere is plentiful—but also often confusing, misleading, or just wrong. My goal in this book is to give you the most up-to-date, accurate, and helpful information I can, drawing on years of experience helping people heal their feet. I want you to understand why a particular treatment is recommended. I want you to understand the basics of home-based therapy and why orthotics (custom or off-the-shelf) may be needed. I want you to spend the least amount of time and money to get the best results. I want you to know the right questions to ask your health-care team, and I want you to understand the answers.

If there's one thing I've learned from treating so many people with plantar fasciitis, it's that every case is different. What works quickly and well for one person may take longer for someone else, or might not work well at all. Healing is very individual and variable and can take up to six months or, in rare cases, years. The important thing to remember is that in almost every case, healing *will* happen. The hardest part of PF treatment is being patient about it.

Managing PF usually takes a combination of approaches. You may need to make some changes, such as losing weight, that aren't quick or easy. They're worth doing not just to help your foot pain, but to improve your overall health. Heel pain decreases your health-related quality of life by reducing your activity level. When I have to tell my patients who run that they need to stop for a while, that makes them very unhappy. I want to help you return to your normal activity level so you don't have a decreased quality of life overall. I want to help you keep active while you heal to reduce your risk of weight gain, depression, and becoming unfit. I don't want you to stop moving, just tweak the way you do it.

THE PROMISE OF THIS BOOK

My goal with this book is to help you understand plantar fasciitis and to treat it so that your pain decreases as much as possible. (I'd love to say that I can cure your PF, but no such cure really exists.) I want to get you back on your feet and keep you there.

Step 1 is to understand the treatment process. The more you understand about why I recommend the treatment steps I do, the more engaged you will be in the process and the more likely you will be to get a better outcome.

Step 2 is to know what to expect at each level of treatment. This will help you be aware of what we're doing and know what you should expect to feel at each level.

Step 3 is to be an active participant in your treatment. Medicine can be very one-sided and passive—the health-care provider tells you what to do without asking for feedback from you, and you of them. I want to educate you to become a more active participant in your treatment by being a more informed patient.

Step 4 is to pick the right footwear for daily home, work, and other activities. The footwear you choose can greatly affect the time it takes to heal. If you're a lawyer in an office and that culture is all about high heels, or if you're a factory worker and you're working in steel-toe boots, or if you work at home and you go barefoot most of the time—all of those things have implications. I want you to understand how those interplay and come up with a solution that works to help get you better. (There's a reason why I see almost twice as many women as men in my practice. High heels are why I have a job.)

Step 5 is learning how to stay active through plantar fasciitis. I don't want people to stop being active because they have foot pain. When you stop moving, you lose the benefits of staying healthy and being active. Your risk factors for all kinds of health problems, such as diabetes, heart disease, and depression, go up. Being able to keep doing the things that you want to do is crucial to your physical and mental health. I want to help you find ways to be able to do things with less pain so that you can continue to enjoy your life.

Step 6 is to spend your money wisely on PF treatment. I want you to understand the best practices for each aspect of treatment. There are twenty different ways to make an orthotic, and some may be more effective than others for plantar fasciitis. In this book, I'll tell you how to get the right orthotic for you.

I wrote this book for the everyday patient, not as a scholarly text. I want you to easily understand what I'm saying and maybe even enjoy reading this book.

HOW COMMON IS PF?

Plantar fasciitis is very common. It's been shown to affect 10 percent of the general population. It also has been shown to affect 10 to 20 percent of runners. Your age affects your risk. Among people over the age of 65, about 7 percent have plantar fasciitis (Cutts et al. 2012). If you have diabetes, you're at greater risk of PF. Even if you don't have any particular risk factors, you can still get PF. I got plantar fasciitis by playing with my son while barefoot. I got up off the ground too quickly, with my toes overextended, and actually tore my plantar fascia. It can happen to people who garden a lot in a kneeling position, with their toes extended back. From Payton Manning in the NFL, to parents playing with their kids, anyone can get it.

There are many ways to get plantar fasciitis. People who aren't that active and then do too much, too soon, too fast in a new activity are likely to get PF. Excess body weight and poor ankle flexibility are two proven risk factors. So are wearing inappropriate footwear and wearing worn-out shoes. Walking and standing on hard surfaces for long periods of time also increases your risk. In other words, PF doesn't strike randomly—there are usually causes for it.

WHY AREN'T YOU GETTING BETTER?

Until recently, the scientific literature on plantar fasciitis said that no evidence strongly supports the effectiveness of any one treatment for plantar fasciitis. Supposedly, most patients just improve on their own over nine or ten months without doing anything. Basically, the literature said to do nothing and it will get better on its own—it can be a self-resolving condition. Unfortunately, that sort of old thinking is still heard today in clinical practice.

People come into my office and say, "My doctor told me to just wait it out, but I haven't been able to be active. I'm getting depressed. I don't feel good; I'm gaining weight." What they're really saying is that their quality of life is going down. Many of my patients get caught in a cascading cycle of pain, reduced activity, continuing pain, even less activity, weight gain, and depression—and pain. What's worse, because they're not getting any treatment at all with conservative therapies, they can wind up with a secondary injury. That's because they change the way they walk to compensate for the plantar fasciitis pain and start getting knee, hip, or back problems. The compensation might even lead to getting plantar fasciitis in the other foot as well.

Medicine is slow to change, even when change is supported by good research. Not everyone on your health-care team may be up on the best evidence to treat your plantar fasciitis. As a foot specialist, I know that there are lots of evidence-based, effective things you can do that can help you get better. This book shows you how to apply them in a logical, algorithm-like fashion.

Different treatments work for different people at different rates. One person is going to get better by doing foot stretches for six weeks. Another is going to need four different therapies that will take six months. Your feet are very complicated—each one has twenty-six bones (twenty-eight if you count the sesamoid bones), plus lots of ligaments, tendons, and muscles. Those bones form a very tightly packed structure, and they move only in very small amounts. That makes it difficult to do accurate biomechanical research. New imaging techniques are just starting to give us better clues as to why things work the way they do in your feet. The research so far hasn't given us a definitive cure for plantar fasciitis. What it has done is help us find better ways to manage the recovery process from start to finish.

INJURY AND RE-INJURY

One of the most frustrating things about PF is that it is a cyclical pattern of retearing and half-healing. That's why you're sore on those first ten or twenty steps and why I'm going to focus a lot on what you can do to help yourself with those first steps in the morning or after you've been sitting for more than twenty minutes. Your foot relaxes while you sleep. The damaged soft tissue starts to half-heal in that relaxed position. Then when you get up and put weight on your feet, your arch lowers, increasing the strain on your plantar fascia (Cutts et al. 2012). The increased strain results in a retearing of the half-healing from the night before, with those first ten steps. In this book, I want to show you how to break up that cycle of half-healing and retearing by giving you evidence-based and clinically proven strategies that reduce your morning symptoms. I'll help you avoid reinjuring yourself every morning and give you a better chance to heal.

I view each of my patients as an individual research project. Because people are variable, they're going to respond variably. Having access to the best research is how we as clinicians make informed decisions, but since most is based on a normally distributed population, that centers around a mean, if you're one of the outliers (and I'd argue that lots of my patients are), then it might not always apply to you. Perhaps, you're the one who will respond differently. What I hope to do in this book is to take over fourteen years of clinical experience treating thousands of cases of plantar fasciitis and combine the best clinical knowledge with the best research. I want to combine what my patients have told me are their expectations with the latest research, and what we know works clinically to help you manage your plantar fasciitis. This is the real definition of evidence-based practice (Sackett 1996). Not just doing what the research alone says. I think we've forgotten that along the way and rely too much only on the research as gospel.

For health-care practitioners, I hope this book will help you understand how to apply evidence-based practices to your patients with PF. I'll give my take on the best available evidence to date—why it might be good, why it might not be so good—and help you find treatment solutions for your patients. This book is designed primarily for patients, so most of this will take place on our companion website, **www.thepfplan.com**.

WHAT'S IN THIS BOOK?

This book is a step-by-step roadmap for getting better. I give you a solid basic understanding of what plantar fasciitis is and then give starting steps for improving. Unless you're a super foot nerd like me, you probably won't read this book cover to cover. I want you to think of it more like a manual than a novel. I hope you'll read chapter 1 so you understand the basics of PF: what it is and why we don't know what we don't know. Then I hope you'll go to the first phase of treatment. If you follow the information there, you may end up 100 percent better within six weeks. That would be awesome. Next, I hope you read the section on prevention, because if you're recovered I want you to stay that way.

If you do the first phase of treatment and it doesn't work completely, move on to Phase 2; move on to Phase 3 only if needed. If you're a non-responder and you need a specialist to re-manage your case, you might say to me, "I've already done some exercises." But were they the best ones given your particular circumstance? You might say, "I've already had orthotics." But were they the right ones, properly designed and fitted? If you've been through ineffective treatment, it's possible that you can still benefit from re-managing your case with a more individual focus. That's what happens with about 15 percent of the people I see. When we take a different approach that combines treatments, they almost always benefit.

Let's get started on getting you out of pain!

PART ONE

SO YOU HAVE THIS PAIN IN YOUR HEEL...

CHAPTER 1

ANATOMY OF PLANTAR FASCIITIS

You've got this pain in your heel, especially first thing in the morning, that just won't go away. What's causing it? You have plantar fasciitis. At its core, plantar fasciitis (PF) is an inflammation of the fascia at your heel—that's what the -*itis* part means. There's lots of academic discussion on the true nature of PF. Some say it's truly inflammation, while others argue that the tissues are degrading. We'll dive deeper into that in later chapters, but for most people, plantar fasciitis means pain on the inside bottom part of your heel, especially when they wake up in the morning. If you don't have pain in the inside bottom part of your heel—if the pain is somewhere else on your foot, like the back part of the heel—it's probably not plantar fasciitis.

The hallmark of plantar fasciitis is pain on the bottom, inside part of your heel after periods of rest. You might be reading this and think, "But most of my pain is at night. What gives?" Don't worry. While the majority of typical cases present with morning pain, some atypical cases hurt only later in the day.

Why does it hurt? Maybe it's inflammation, maybe it's tissue degradation, or perhaps even both. The experts all admit that the cause of plantar fasciitis isn't clearly understood. Whatever the cause, managing the problem is easier if you understand a little bit about the anatomy of your foot and what the plantar fascia actually is.

WHAT IS YOUR PLANTAR FASCIA?

The plantar fascia is a flat band of dense connective tissue that connects your heel bone to your toes. Plantar is the anatomical term for the sole of your foot; fascia is the anatomical term for band. The plantar fascia starts at the bottom of your heel and ends at the ball of your foot. While the plantar fascia shares characteristics with tendons (connective tissue that attaches muscles to bones) and ligaments (connective tissue that connect bones), its function is to support the arch of the foot and keep it structurally stable.

The overall structural stability of your foot comes primarily by the way all the pieces fit tightly together. The bones, the ligaments, the

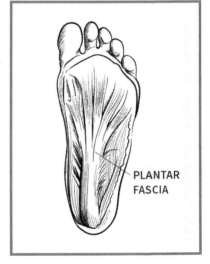

PLANTAR FASCIA

tendons, and the muscles all provide shape and support, but the plantar fascia has the greatest effect on overall foot integrity. If your plantar fascia is cut, you lose 25 percent of the stability in the foot (Huang et al. 1993).

A famous podiatrist named Dr. Kevin Kirby has suggested the main functions of the plantar fascia (Kirby 2016). According to Dr. Kirby, your plantar fascia:

- Supports the medial (inside) and lateral (outside) longitudinal arches of your foot—it gives them their shape and structure.
- Aids in making your foot more efficient when you go to push off as you take a step.
- Assists the lower leg muscles by eliminating movement at the foot and assists the deep muscles in your foot in preventing arch flattening.
- Reduces forces on the ligaments on the bottom part of your foot.
- Prevents excessive compression on the joints in the top of your foot.
- Prevents excessive bending stress on the metatarsals (toe bones).
- Allows you to keep your toes on the ground and helps stabilize your toes.
- Reduces forces on the small bones at the ball of your foot on the bottom.
- Helps to absorb and release elastic energy during running and jumping activities.

The broad band of connective tissue that is the plantar fascia provides a strong mechanical linkage between the heel and the toes. It provides linkages into muscles, the supporting structures in the bottom part of your foot, and even the skin itself. The plantar fascia starts at the inside part of the heel and fans out to run across the sole of your foot in three bands: medial, or the inside part of your foot; central; and lateral, or the outside part of your foot. It's interesting to note that the plantar fascia is somewhat variable. The medial and lateral bands can differ in size and thickness. In about 12 percent of people, the lateral band isn't even there (Wearing et al. 2006).

In plantar fasciitis, clinically, I find most people are the most tender on both the medial and the central band of their plantar fascia. When I push along that tissue on the bottom part of the foot, they're more sensitive toward the inside and the middle part of their arch. That's because most people pronate when they walk—they put more pressure on the inside of their foot than the outside of their foot. I think that ends up putting a mechanical strain on the tissue on the middle inside more than the middle outside.

People often mistakenly think the plantar fascia is a continuation of the Achilles tendon. That's because the Achilles tendon is the attachment point at the heel bone for the calf muscles in the back part of the leg. Because it's in close proximity to the plantar fascia, people think that it wraps around the heel or that it's a continuation of the calf muscles. Research has shown that the plantar fascia develops independently and that in adults it is entirely separate from the Achilles tendon (Snow et al. 1995). In fact, if you damage your Achilles tendon, it would be unlikely to affect the plantar fascia, unless you change the way you walk.

Ninety percent or more of people with plantar fasciitis experience pain in the heel itself. To understand why, let's look at how the plantar fascia is attached to the medial calcaneus, or heel bone. The connective tissue that attaches directly to the bone is called the fibrocartilage. This junction has four zones that range from bone to really, really stiff connective tissue, to soft tissue (Wearing et al. 2006). The zone arrangement allows for a greater dispersion of force when your heel hits the ground (Wearing et al. 2006). It also lets your foot better resist movement from multiple directions. If you're playing tennis, for instance, you're putting a lot of side-to-side and back-and-forth pressure on your foot. The zone arrangement evens out the load. The plantar fascia tissue itself is actually relatively inelastic, so it helps hold your foot in place.

The pain of plantar fasciitis is felt in the heel at and around the point where the fascia originates from the heel bone. That's the point of greatest impact whenever you take a step, so that's the point that gets irritated the most. But what have you done to make your foot hurt? That's what I'll explain in the next chapter.

CHAPTER 2

CAUSES

W hat causes plantar fasciitis? That's probably the question I hear most from my patients. The real question is, what is the best current understanding of what causes plantar fasciitis? Our best understanding is that when some kind of a stressor disrupts the attachment point of the plantar fascia at the heel bone, things start to go wrong. But what causes the disruption? The simple answer to that is there's no one way to get PF.

Lots of predisposing factors could cause irritation to that site. Sometimes it's too much, too soon, too fast of an activity. Or it could be running in shoes that are worn-out, or footwear that doesn't fit properly or is inappropriate for your activity, or standing on hard surfaces for long periods of time. It could be that you've gained some extra weight recently, or it could be a combination of factors—anything that puts stress on the bottom of the foot at the heel. Anything that overextends the plantar fascia, such as kneeling and digging your toes into the ground while gardening, can also damage it. And as we age and enter our forties, the fat pad underneath the plantar fascia starts to thin, which puts more strain on the attachment point and makes damage easier. As we reach age sixty plus, the plantar fascia becomes more brittle and more prone to injury.

Whatever the predisposing factor, you're creating microtraumas—microscopic tears—in the fascia. The tears cause inflammation, which is your body's normal response to damage. Inflammation causes pain, swelling, and reduced function. We can think of this as the acute phase of PF.

After the initial factor causes some type of change and micro-trauma, if it doesn't resolve during the acute stage, the plantar fascia itself starts to degenerate and get stiffer (Wearing et al. 2006). That will increase the strain and tension at the attachment point to the heel bone. This degeneration may or may not be accompanied by inflammation and pain as your body tries to repair the damage. On top of this is the cycle of half-healing and re-injury, which only makes things worse.

Interestingly, not every case of plantar fasciitis shows signs of inflammation. Those cases make us think that perhaps fasciitis isn't the right term. Remember, -itis means inflammation. In people who have chronic plantar fasciitis, however, we don't see inflammation markers. For those people, a better way to think of the condition might be as plantar fasciosis (Wearing et al. 2006). The -osis suffix means an ongoing condition that gradually degrades the tissue. It's possible that inflammation and degradation could actually represent two different but coexisting problems in the foot!

Most plantar fasciitis is caused by microtrauma, but it's possible for your plantar fascia to snap suddenly. As we age, increased mineralization of the fibrocartilage at the origin point of the fascia, on the heel, causes it to become more brittle (Wearing et al. 2006). With added mechanical strain, your plantar fascia could rupture. It might happen as an acute injury. I've seen cases where the patient was playing basketball and landed on his foot the wrong way. The landing overstrained the fascia and ruptured it. In those situations, the person usually hears an actual pop as the rupture occurs. On the other hand, you can rupture your plantar fascia without any specific injury.

At the end of the day, mechanical overload of the attachment area is thought to be one element in a multifactorial puzzle that can cause degradation overall. Mechanical loading alone isn't always enough, however. It's possible that poor blood flow combines with mechanical strain to cause irritation. The plantar fascia, like other tough connective tissues in the body, is poorly vascularized—it just doesn't have a lot of blood vessels. That could be one of the reasons we see more plantar fasciitis in people who have complications of diabetes. Their blood flow to the small vessels of the feet is usually compromised, which limits the blood flow to the plantar fascia even more. When people with diabetes get peripheral neuropathy (a lowering of the ability of the sensory nerves in the feet to work properly) from nerve damage in the feet, they may have balance problems that affect the way they walk. These imbalances and gait changes can stretch and damage the plantar fascia.

Tissue degradation in plantar fasciitis is basically the destruction of the collagen fibers in the dense connective tissue that makes up the fascia. Collagen is the body's main structural protein—it's what holds us together. When collagen in the plantar fascia starts to break down, that's when things really start to go awry, as the plantar fascia starts to degrade. Ordinarily, the collagen fibers are ropey—they should be long and tightly packed. When they start to break down, they get loose and disarranged. When that happens, plantar fasciitis can become chronic and take a long time to heal.

In the early stages of PF, we try to decrease inflammation and break up the cycle of half-healing and retearing. If you don't respond to that, then we try to do things like off-load the tissue and keep it in a lengthened position that allows those collagen fibers to start aligning themselves better. When tissue degradation starts, we can stop it in most people, but it can take a long time.

IS IT REALLY PLANTAR FASCIITIS?

Not all pain in the bottom part of your heel is plantar fasciitis. Other structures in that area could be causing the discomfort. It could be fat pad syndrome, which is a breakdown of the fat pad underneath your heel. That would cause pain because the cushioning it provides is no longer there. It might be bursitis. There's a small bursa underneath the point where the plantar fascia attaches to the heel itself. A bursa is a small, fluid-filled sac that acts as cushion. Sometimes that bursa becomes inflamed, causing pain. In rare cases, the pain is caused by an illness such as rheumatoid arthritis or fibromyalgia. Osteoarthritis doesn't cause heel pain per se, but it can stiffen the joints in the foot and leg. When the joints aren't moving well, that could produce strain on the soft tissues that would lead to PF. Nerve entrapment can also mask itself as plantar fasciitis, causing severe pain in the heel. Bottom line? See your primary care physician or a sport and exercise medicine physician who can accurately diagnose your pain. (I'm not that kind of doctor. I like to say that I'm the kind of doctor they let into the research lab but not the medicine cabinet.)

HEEL SPURS

A heel spur is a bony projection from the back or bottom of the calcaneus (heel bone) that can make walking painful. Many people have heel spurs that don't cause pain—to be exact, painless heel spurs occur in 15 to 40 percent of adults (Michelsson et al. 2005). In fact, they might not even know they have them unless they get their foot X-rayed for some other reason. A painful heel spur on the bottom of the foot is usually the *result* of plantar fasciitis, not

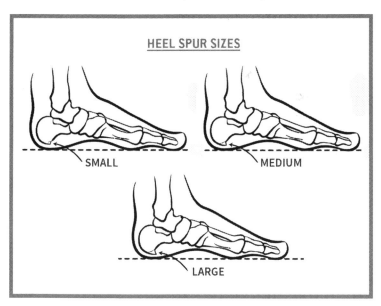

HEEL SPUR SIZES

SMALL   MEDIUM

LARGE

necessarily the cause of it, but you can have painful heel spurs without plantar fasciitis. No matter the cause, heel spur pain can be different from PF pain. Much as PF may be the combination of inflammation and degeneration, heel spurs and plantar fasciitis can coexist. In a normal case of PF, you have pain when you take your first steps after resting, especially first thing in the morning. Heel spurs often don't usually hurt when you wake up. Rather, they hurt after you've been on your feet for a longer period of time. If you have no pain when you wake up first thing in the morning but do have pain with cumulative time on your feet, that can mean you have atypical PF, painful heel spurs, or perhaps something else.

How does PF cause heel spurs? As your plantar fascia stiffens, it increases the tensile force at the attachment point on the heel. To cope with the stress, your body remodels the bone around the area, which is what actually produces the heel spurs. One theory suggests that heel spurs develop as a protective mechanism to keep the PF from bending as much, thus reducing strain. Depending on the size of the heel spur, the spur itself can cause entrapment of one of the small nerves at the bottom of the foot, such as the lateral plantar nerve, and that can give you symptoms similar to plantar fasciitis (Chundru et al. 2008). You'll feel pain and a burning sensation in the area innervated by the nerve itself. Long-term compression of those nerves can actually cause muscle wasting in the bottom part of the foot (Chundru et al. 2008). That can lead to a downward spiral where the muscles atrophy and no longer provide adequate strength and stability. Over time, your foot weakens, which can lead to a reoccurrence of plantar fasciitis. It is also important to note that the length of the heel spur has been shown to correlate with an increase in pain and decreased functional scores in patients with PF (Kuyucu et al. 2015).

Even if you have a heel spur, surgeons do not typically remove or perform surgery for it. Treatment of painful heel spurs may include orthotics (off-the-shelf or custom) similar to those used for plantar fasciitis, where the goal is to remove pressure from the painful area.

CHAPTER 3

SYMPTOMS

The hallmark symptom of plantar fasciitis is pain on the bottom, inside part of your heel after periods of rest. People describe the pain in a variety of different ways. It could be sharp; it could be dull; it could be achy; it could be burning. It could be all of those things. The quality of pain differs in how people describe it, but the location is usually the same.

Plantar fasciitis is often most painful right after you wake up in the morning and take your first ten to twenty steps. If you have PF, that's usually the worst part of your day. You've rested for the longest period of the day while you slept. At night while you sleep, your foot relaxes. All the damaged soft tissue starts to half-heal in this relaxed and shortened position. Then, when you get up and put weight on your foot, your arch lowers, and you increase the stretch on your plantar fascia. That increases the tensile pulling on the attachment point at the heel. With every step, you're retearing the half-healing from the night before. That's where a lot of the pain comes from, so that's the most important part to pay attention to.

The pain usually improves after the first ten to twenty steps because now you've re-torn the tissue to the point where you can walk on it with a baseline level of pain. This is why some people can often be active with plantar fasciitis, and it doesn't cause any problems *while* they're in motion. If they sit down for a while and then get up again, the pain gets worse because the tissue starts to try to heal again.

Some of my patients are in so much pain they tell me they literally crawl to the bathroom in the morning because they can't stand on their foot. Others say that it's particularly bad after a rest period. The amount of pain differs greatly. Some people just can't function with their first ten steps. They describe walking down the stairs sideways so they don't have to put pressure on their heel. They describe walking on their toes or their forefoot only because they're not able to put pressure on their heel. Once their foot "warms up," they feel better. What some people think is that taking those first ten steps is actually doing them good. They think that they feel better after those steps because they've warmed up their foot. What they don't realize is that it's exactly the opposite. When you take those ten steps, that's when you're doing the most damage for the rest of the day. That's counterintuitive. People don't always associate the damage they're doing with the ongoing pain. When I explain it to them, it's as if a light bulb goes off in their heads. It's always best to stay off any injury. Once they realize that their PF really is an injury, they understand why the first step in treatment is not to walk on the foot first thing in the morning.

What people usually tell me is that it hurts first thing in the morning. It hurts when they've been in their car for twenty minutes and get back out again. It hurts when they go home at the end of the day and sit down, watch some TV, read a book, and go to get back up again. It typically hurts more barefoot than when they are in shoes. Wearing footwear around the house makes them feel better. Most people are sore in the morning and evening and can manage during the day. It just depends on how bad their plantar fasciitis is. With mild plantar fasciitis, you might only have pain with your first ten steps in the morning, and it might be only low-grade pain. You might not even have pain after prolonged rest. If you have moderate to severe plantar fasciitis, it's going to hurt when you sit down for ten minutes and go to get up again. It's going to feel like someone's sticking an ice pick in the bottom part of your foot.

Because I'm a pedorthist who treats people with orthotics and footwear, my patients have usually been suffering with PF for a while before they see me. Because I don't believe custom-made orthotics (inserts that go in your shoes) are the first line of treatment for acute PF, my patients have tried a lot of other solutions first. I don't typically see them until things such as staying off their foot for a little bit hasn't worked, and they've gone on to do physiotherapy and taken a round of medications. When all of those things haven't worked, then they come to see me.

The reason I'm writing this book is because I see so many people whose PF hasn't been managed that well, mostly because there's a general lack of understanding about the condition. Whenever we try to fit simplistic answers to complex questions, they usually don't work. I feel that if most of my patients had followed my Phase I (REST) program from the start, they might have had a better chance of getting better and never needed to come see me at all. Yes, I wrote this in the hopes that more people wouldn't have to see me! (Somewhere there's a business consultant who just had a mild heart episode.)

Therapists differ in their approach to treatment for plantar fasciitis. Some of my patients were given foot stretches to do. That's the right idea, but they were given the wrong stretches—the ones that have been proven to be less effective compared to the targeted set I usually recommend, based on the evidence. I want people to be better-educated consumers when they go for therapy. One problem is that not all therapists have the specialized knowledge about PF to give you the right exercises. The same is true for orthotics. Many of the professionals who provide them just don't know as much as they could about plantar fasciitis. They design orthotics that may not be as effective as they should be. They don't have the knowledge to explain to you why you need to change your footwear and do the Phase 1 exercises first thing in the morning.

Some of my patients have faithfully followed the exercises they were told to do and actually made things worse. I'll go into this in much more detail in chapter 7, but for now, it's important to know that there are two different kinds of exercises you can do for plantar fasciitis. Most people are told to do the generic calf stretches up against a wall. My patients are told to do tissue-specific exercises before they even take a step in the morning. The problem with the generic approach is that you do it once you're already up and walking around.

People come in to my clinic and say, "Oh yeah, I was given some stretches to do up against the wall."

I say, "Great, when do you do them?"

They say, "Well, I'll get up. I'll go have a shower. I'll get dressed, and then I'll do my stretches and go to work." At that point, you've already gone through your first twenty steps and then some before you even think about your stretches, which means you've already done the damage for the rest of the day. Remember, we need to break the cycle!

If you don't have pain in the morning, you probably don't have a typical case of plantar fasciitis. The same is true if your feet get worse the more you're on them all day. If your feet hurt more the longer you're on them, that typically isn't a sign of plantar fasciitis. It's more likely to be bursitis or a heel spur or maybe a fat pad problem. On the other hand, if you have an acute case of PF, everything is going to hurt you. You might also have atypical symptoms of plantar fasciitis, such as pain in the front of your arch. Your plantar fascia runs from its origin on the heel up into the toes. The biggest insertions are basically at the ball of the foot. Some people will have no pain at the heel, but they'll have pain at the ball of the foot where the plantar fascia inserts around the metatarsal heads (toe bones). When you bend the toes back and increase the tensile load to the fascia and then press on it, you get lots of pain. Atypical cases of plantar fasciitis are relatively rare—I estimate they make up only about 5 percent of the cases I see.

CHAPTER 4

RISK FACTORS

A lthough plantar fasciitis often seems to happen out of the blue, in fact, most people who get it have some risk factors. Some, like the shoes you wear, can be controlled or avoided. Some, like injuries and the shape of the arch in your foot, can't.

FOOTWEAR

In my opinion, bad footwear can definitely cause plantar fasciitis. I think of footwear in three different ways: you fit the individual shoe for the foot, you fit the shoe to the person's individual biomechanics, and then you fit the shoe to the particular activity that person's going to be doing.

Getting the correct size shoe is essential. If your shoes are too big or too small, that makes you curl up your toes more or it makes your foot shift more in the shoe. Both can affect your PF.

If you buy the wrong type of shoe for the mechanical profile of your foot, that can put stress and strain on the bottom of your foot and irritate the attachment point for the plantar fascia at the heel. For example, if you're a supinator—your foot rolls to the outside when you take a step—and you buy a stability shoe that pushes you even further to the outside, the stress and strain can lead to PF.

If you're wearing the incorrect shoe for the type of activity that you're doing, you're at risk for PF. For instance, if you go for a long walk in flip-flops instead of hiking boots or running shoes, that can definitely cause a repetitive strain on the bottom part of your foot.

How old is your footwear? Some of the people who come to me for PF treatment are wearing shoes where the heel is so worn that it's almost at a 45-degree angle—seriously, take a look at some of the pictures. They've worn the shoe halfway through the midsole, and now it's forcing them to walk in a distorted way that's straining their plantar fascia. I see a lot of people who decided on the first nice spring day that they'd go out for a run. They dug out their old running shoes from the back of the closet, dusted them off, and started their run without noticing that the shoes were worn-out and should really have been replaced. They do a couple of runs, and all of a sudden, they have foot pain. Old, worn-out shoes are a risk factor for PF. Old, worn-out shoes plus carrying extra weight is an even bigger risk factor. In my view, you're basically asking to get hurt. We'll touch on all of this and when to replace your footwear in chapter 9.

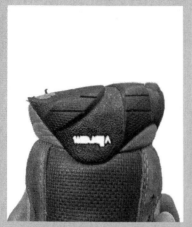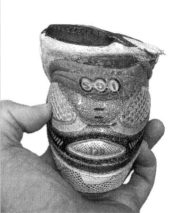

Shoes that have been worn well past their lifetime—notice the angle the shoe is now on.

Increased loading under the heel may be a risk factor for plantar fasciitis. The more load your heel takes with every step, the more likely you are to develop plantar fasciitis. In men's dress shoes, for instance, wearing really hard, leather-soled shoes and standing for excessive periods of time increases the load at the heel. I see a lot of university professors and other professionals who stand for long periods of time in those traditional, hard leather dress shoes. Conversely, women who have plantar fasciitis and wear high heels often find that the heels reduce some of their symptoms. That's because the heels move the load from your heel, but you just end up putting it somewhere else that can get sore, which is the ball of your foot.

The interesting thing about running shoes when it comes to injury prevention is that even though there have been huge strides recently in materials engineering and footwear engineering to make a better shoe, injury rates in runners keep going up. I can tell you from my years of experience that when you wear the wrong shoes, that's when you're likely to develop plantar fasciitis.

I'll go into detail about choosing appropriate footwear for different activities in chapter 10.

HIGH AND LOW ARCHES

The arch of your foot transfers your body weight from your heel to your toes when you take a step. Some people naturally have low arches—the height of the arch is below average. You can see this if your footprint while you're barefoot shows most of the bottom of your foot. There's been a lot of research trying to show that a low-arched foot is a risk factor or even a causative factor for plantar fasciitis. That link still hasn't been conclusively shown, because there are lots of people who have low-arched feet and don't have plantar fasciitis. Some of the studies show a correlation between low arches and plantar fasciitis, but correlation doesn't mean causation. (At last, I can use something from my second-year statistics class!) What we can say, based on the research, is that if you have low arches and plantar fasciitis, your low arches may or may not have caused your plantar fasciitis, but they can play a role in why you're not getting better (Wearing et al. 2004).

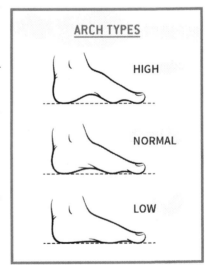

ARCH TYPES

HIGH

NORMAL

LOW

Intuitively, we look at flat feet and say, "Oh my gosh, look at those things. Of course they're going to cause problems." In fact, there's no good scientific evidence to suggest that flat feet are the causative factor of injury. Doing things, such as orthotics, preventatively for flat feet hasn't yet been proven to be definitively effective. There is, however, some evidence in runners that choosing footwear to better stabilize a flatter foot may reduce the likelihood of injury (Malisoux et al. 2016).

When we look at the opposite situation, in a higher-arched foot, we see a foot that's more inflexible, more immobile, doesn't absorb shock very well, and doesn't accommodate to changes in surface very well. Research estimates that up to 60 percent of people with high-arched feet will experience *chronic* foot pain (Burns et al. 2007). People with high arches are more likely to develop PF and other injuries under the ball of the foot (Burns et al. 2007). We can actually do preventative things with orthotics and footwear for higher-arched feet. These techniques can reduce foot pain up to 75 percent (Burns et al. 2007).

The height of your arch is simply the way you are. I like to think about people on a continuum, because it elegantly answers the clinical question: How can some people be so low-arched that their full arch touches the ground like a flat pancake, but they can run marathons pain free? And how can people who have relatively small deviations from "normal" biomechanics have a ton of pain and problems?

What it comes down to in my mind is a theory of injury proposed in the 1990s called soft tissue stress theory (McPoil and Hunt

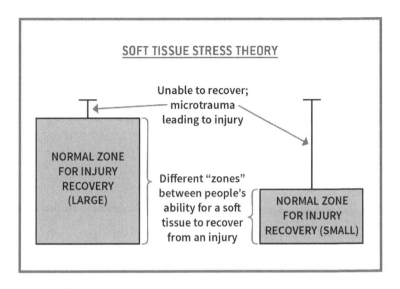

SOFT TISSUE STRESS THEORY

Unable to recover; microtrauma leading to injury

NORMAL ZONE FOR INJURY RECOVERY (LARGE)

Different "zones" between people's ability for a soft tissue to recover from an injury

NORMAL ZONE FOR INJURY RECOVERY (SMALL)

1995). The theory basically says that you can treat a soft tissue in the body like a materials engineering problem. Some people can subject their soft tissues to repetitive stress within a large zone (see the image that follows), where they're able to naturally recover. Other people naturally have a very small zone for their soft tissue to take repetitive stress, meaning that their upper and lower boundaries are very narrow (McPoil and Hunt 1995). They're always going to have a greater chance of being injured. That's why someone with a normal-looking foot can be plagued with problems and pain. (You can watch me explain this concept in person at **thepfplan.com/videos**.)

Everybody is different. Your foot has so many bones, tendons, ligaments, and muscles that it's surprising more doesn't go wrong. The individual variability with how all these elements interact is huge. There are twenty-six bones in the foot, and the way those bones touch each other and articulate with one another is different for everybody. Some people just have larger joint ranges of motion; some people just have smaller ones. Some people have no range of motion—those bones are actually fused together. What scares me is when we try to make one answer fit everybody.

HARD SURFACES

Prolonged standing and walking on hard surfaces, such as the concrete floors in a warehouse or the linoleum floors in a hospital, is a big risk factor for plantar fasciitis. In one interesting study of male factory workers, the researchers found that increased time spent standing on hard surfaces increased the risk of plantar fasciitis (Werner et al. 2010). As little as a 10 percent increase in the time spent walking on hard floors increased the risk of plantar fasciitis in the group studied by 52 percent (Werner et al. 2010). The study controlled for other factors that are associated with PF, such as being overweight, and still found that the time spent standing and walking on hard surfaces was closely correlated to the chances of getting plantar fasciitis. Another significant risk factor was the number of times they got in and out of their forklift or truck in a given day. Rotating their footwear between at least two different types of shoes decreased the incidence of plantar fasciitis by 72 percent (Werner et al. 2010). I would suggest that time allowed the softer materials in the boot's midsole the opportunity to rebound and to continue to provide cushioning. We make the same footwear rotation suggestion to runners who run on consecutive days.

I see a lot of nurses who have plantar fasciitis from spending twelve-hour shifts on hospital floors, which are usually linoleum over concrete. I also see a lot of teachers, because they're on their feet for long periods of time as well.

Hard floors just don't have any give, which increases the loading rate underneath the heel. Studies show us that the more loading that happens underneath the heel, the more likely you are to develop plantar fasciitis. It's not the work itself that's causing PF in these people; it may be the surface they do the work on.

One study alone may not tell the entire story, though. A systematic review in 2015 concluded that due to the small number of studies done on the topic (only four met the criteria), and questions as to the quality of the research that currently exists, more research is needed before being able to fully determine the relationship between work surfaces and PF (Waclawski et al. 2015). Don't give up your day just yet!

TIGHT MUSCLES

Can you extend your leg and easily point your toes back toward your ankle? That's called dorsiflexion. (Pointing your toes down, away from your ankle, is called plantarflexion.) If you have a reduction in dorsiflexion of the ankle, it usually comes from tight calf muscles. Bone deformity and injury can also reduce dorsiflexion. Reduced dorsiflexion can be a mechanical determinant in plantar fasciitis (Bolívar et al. 2013). The reason is a little complex. For you to be able to walk, your body has to get your leg over the top of your foot. That sounds simple, but if you have biomechanical abnormalities that don't allow that to happen easily, you have to compensate. When you have inadequate dorsiflexion, you still have to get your body forward somehow. Your foot is going to make compensations to allow you to do that. One way is to out-toe your foot, which causes you to pronate more (roll in your foot). When you out-toe and pronate, you put more load on your plantar fascia. Another way to compensate is to lift your heel up off the ground sooner than you typically would. Again, that increases strain on your plantar fascia. Some people will do a combination of compensations. It all leads to more mechanical loading of the plantar fascia and a greater risk of the damage that causes PF.

In one study, after controlling for other factors such as weight, gender, and age, tight hamstrings were shown to have a greater association (8.7 times as likely) in people who have plantar fasciitis (Labovitz and Yu 2011). Muscle tightness can be caused by inactivity, injury, or inadequate stretching after activity (not cooling down properly), and even sleeping posture. And some people just have tight hamstrings and aren't very flexible naturally. When you have tight hamstrings, the muscles in the back part of your upper legs get tight. That makes you contract your calf muscles sooner, which ends up restricting ankle dorsiflexion, which ends up putting more mechanical strain on your plantar fascia.

INJURIES

Any sort of injury that leads to compensation in your gait is a risk factor for PF. If you have a knee injury, for instance, you might be limping around for a few weeks and putting excess load on the other foot, straining the plantar fascia. If another area of your foot hurts and you start to compensate, that can cause plantar fasciitis. If you have a neuroma (a benign growth of nerve tissue, usually between the third and fourth toes), for instance, you have pain between the toes and in the ball of your foot. To compensate, you change your gait to put more weight on your heel. If you have osteoarthritis in your big toe, that makes you walk differently. Any sort of injury from the hip down is going to change your gait and strain the soft tissues more.

ACTIVITY AND OVERUSE INJURIES

I always see a big influx of plantar fasciitis cases in January— Christmas comes a month late for me! Why? New Year's resolutions. Someone resolves to run every day, even though he or she hasn't run at all since his or her last New Year's resolution. They do too much, too soon, too fast and end up in my office with plantar fasciitis. The same thing happens in the early spring when people start riding their bikes again and hurt their knees, which then leads to stress of the plantar fascia from gait compensation. And then there's sandal season. In the summertime, people get out of their regular shoes and start wearing flip-flops. Sometimes this drastic change can lead to PF.

A friend of mine is a sales rep who doesn't have a lot of time to be active or be with his family. He called me one day and said, "Hey, my foot's getting kind of sore."

> I said, "What happened?"
> He said, "I've been doing these super dad runs. I'll send you a picture."

The picture he sent showed him running while carrying one kid on his back and pushing the other kid in a stroller. No surprise that he developed PF.

Changes in your work can be behind PF. If you switch to a job that's way more physically demanding, you're in a too-much,

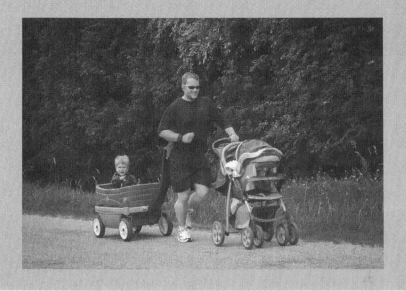

too-soon, too-fast situation. The average person takes between five and ten thousand steps a day. If you suddenly move to a job that makes you take fifteen thousand steps a day, or involves a lot of squatting down and getting up, that can produce more strain on the bottom of your foot.

Your athletic activities give you a lot of ways to get plantar fasciitis. There's poor technique, training errors, too high intensity, and training while you're fatigued. Repetitive loading, muscle dysfunction, and inflexibility can all work to contribute to plantar fasciitis (Beeson 2014).

AGING

Another factor that can cause plantar fasciitis is simply getting older. We see more PF in older athletes, for example. Age-related degenerative changes may result in the fascia's inability to resist normal tensile loads. As we get older, all our tissues become a little stiffer. When you take the already inelastic tissue of the plantar fascia and make it even more inelastic, the pull at the origin point at the heel is increased. At the same time, once we reach age forty, the fat pad underneath the heel starts to thin. The protective mechanisms that protect against shock and loading start to work less well. That increases your risk for PF.

YOUR WEIGHT

Being overweight or obese simply puts more mechanical load on the feet, which can lead to microtrauma that then causes PF. Carrying excess weight also compresses the fat pad under the heel and makes it lose elasticity. When that protective mechanism is compromised, the risk of PF goes up. Many overweight people also have prediabetes or diabetes. Plantar fasciitis is more common in people with diabetes.

According to the 2012–2013 Canadian Health Measures Survey, almost two out of every three Canadians aged eighteen to seventy-nine are overweight or obese based on their body mass index (BMI). (Your BMI is a measure of body fat based on your height and weight. The normal range for BMI is eighteen to twenty-four; to find your BMI, use a chart such as the one found at bmicalculatorcanada.com.) In other words, 62 percent of the adult population is overweight or obese; only 36 percent have a normal BMI. According to the 2009–2012 National Health and Nutrition Examination Survey (NHANES), in the United States, more than two-thirds (68.7 percent) of adults aged twenty and up are overweight or obese; 6.3 percent are extremely obese. Only about 25 percent of the population is normal weight or underweight.

What's even scarier is that 31.8 percent of youth are either over-weight or obese; 16.9 percent of youth are obese. The collective health-care costs of those diagnosed as obese in the United States is some $174 billion a year.

It's clear that we're heavier than ever as a population. We know plantar fasciitis is directly affected by weight—the higher your BMI, the greater your risk. Currently, PF affects about 10 percent of the population. If we don't collectively change weight for the better, I fear that number will rise.

Nutrition experts are beginning to have new conversations around the outdated idea that fat makes you fat. In fact, sugar, from the simple form found in sodas and sweets to processed starchy carbohydrates (breads, pasta, baked goods, snack foods, etc.) may have a more direct role in our expanding waistlines. In his bestselling book *Wheat Belly*, William Davis, MD, makes a great argument for the role of processed wheat in the expansion of our bellies. He suggests that the "accumulation of fat is the result of years of consuming foods containing wheat that triggers insulin, the fat-storing hormone." Dr. Davis goes on to suggest that there is hardly a body system unaffected negatively by the consumption of wheat. In his cardiology practice, he has seen the reversal of heart disease and type 2 diabetes from cutting wheat out of the diet. He has also seen significant weight loss (up to fifty-six pounds in six months) with no calorie counting or denial, simply by eliminating wheat. On a personal note, lower-ing my consumption of wheat, in combination with some of the principles I learned from Precision Nutrition, helped me lose forty-five pounds with minimal exercise. Needless to say, I'm a huge fan of Dr. Davis's work and message. (As a reminder here, I'm not a nutritionist, and this isn't professional advice.)

GENDER

The literature on plantar fasciitis is very inconsistent on the role of gender. Some studies claim women are more prone to it; some say men are more prone to it. About two-thirds of my patients are women, but I'm not sure women are more prone to PF. I think I see more women because men are just less likely to seek treatment when their feet hurt. They tough it out instead.

In general, people are slow to seek help for foot pain. Some seek help after a few weeks, while others can take months before they see their physician. I think people have this common misconception that our feet should just hurt. Until it gets really bad, you don't do anything about it. I really want to help people get past that idea; because we know that the earlier you seek treatment for plantar fasciitis, the better you're going to do.

PREGNANCY

Pregnant women are at risk for PF. It's not just that they're carrying extra weight. Pregnant women actually go through changes in their foot structure (Segal et al. 2013). The changes are usually at their worst during a first pregnancy. At a minimum, lots of pregnant women go up half a shoe size; the change can be as great as a size and a half. The same thing happens with subsequent pregnancies, although usually to a lesser extent.

In addition to an increase in weight, it has been suggested that the change is caused by the hormone relaxin (Segal et al. 2013). This is the hormone that relaxes the ligaments of the pelvis and lets it open up for childbirth. Relaxin promotes collagen breakdown. During pregnancy, it may relax the ligaments in your feet, which when combined with the extra weight puts strain on the plantar fascia, especially at the attachment point at the heel. Even when a woman isn't pregnant, the body produces relaxin, and it ebbs and flows throughout the monthly cycle.

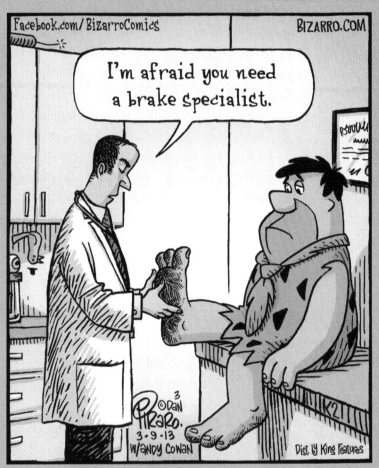

Reprinted with permission of Dan Piraro.

CHAPTER 5

DIAGNOSING

If you have foot pain, diagnosing it quickly and accurately will go a long way toward getting over it quickly. I urge anyone with foot pain that lasts more than four or five days to see a health-care professional quickly. This is even more important if you have diabetes, rheumatoid arthritis, or any other chronic condition, because preexisting conditions can complicate your treatment. If you suspect plantar fasciitis based on what you've already read, it's still important to confirm your self-diagnosis with the professional opinion of your primary care physician.

A good starting point for diagnosis is your primary care physician. However, if you're athletically active, you might want to see a sport and exercise medicine specialist or sport medicine doctor. A primary care foot specialist, such as a chiropodist or a podiatrist, would also be a good option. You wouldn't come to see me for a diagnosis, because I'm a pedorthist with a PhD, not an MD. While I treat PF, I do not diagnose it.

EMERGENCIES

If you've had an acute injury to your foot or ankle, the sort of thing that makes the area swell up or turn black and blue, get to a doctor quickly. For instance, if you have an ankle sprain and you're also worried that you've torn or ruptured your plantar fascia, get it checked. If you felt a large snap or pop, or if it felt like someone hit you in the heel with a baseball bat, and your foot is hurting, go to your doctor or the emergency room as soon as you can. You may have seriously damaged the plantar fascia or something else.

SPECIALISTS

Plantar fasciitis is mostly diagnosed by its clinical symptoms. Your doctor will ask you questions such as the following: Do you have pain in the morning? Do you have pain after rest? The doctor might also palpate your foot to see where the pain is.

Your doctor may send you for an X-ray to see if you have a heel spur and to decide whether or not that could be a contributing factor to your plantar fasciitis. If your recovery doesn't go as well as you hoped and your progress is plateauing, then you might be sent for a diagnostic ultrasound. This has been proven effective for ruling out things such as small tears or even full-thickness tears of the plantar fascia. Ultrasound is relatively low cost and doesn't expose you to any radiation. In general, other imaging tests, such as CT and MRI scans, aren't usually necessary.

TALKING TO YOUR DOCTOR

Because I'm not a primary care provider, I've asked my friend and colleague Tatiana Jevremovic, MD, CCFP(EM), dip sport med sport and exercise medicine physician, to discuss the top-five questions to ask your physician. Here's what she recommends you ask when you visit your doctor to discuss your diagnosis and management of plantar fasciitis.

1. Could this be something else?

Other conditions that can present similarly to plantar fasciitis include plantar fascial tear or fibrosis, fat pad injury, calcaneal stress fracture, and plantar nerve entrapment.

2. Do we need any further investigations?

Plantar fasciitis is a clinical diagnosis most of the time, but certain investigations may be warranted to rule out other pathologies, such as X-ray, ultrasound, bone scan, and MRI.

3. Should I take time off work or modify my duties at work?

If you are on your feet a lot at work, this may slow down or delay your recovery. Exploring your options with your employer is always good (see chapter 19 for more on this).

4. What are the pros and cons of a cortisone injection?

Cortisone can be beneficial in plantar fasciitis, but does have some potential drawbacks. Make sure you discuss this thoroughly. The same question about benefits versus drawbacks should be asked of all other treatment options.

5. What can I do to prevent this from happening again?

Some of the options are discussed in this book (weight loss, proper range of motion, orthotics, and others), but you should always discuss this with your physician to assess your physical readiness.

PART TWO

TREATMENT PHASE 1: HOW TO REST AND RECOVER

MANAGING YOUR PLANTAR FASCIITIS

REST to Break the Pain Cycle

If you have heel pain that's especially bad first thing in the morning or after resting, chances are good you have plantar fasciitis (PF). Removing activity is often recommended as the treatment for PF, but that's not an answer. The rest of this book tells you why and what you can do to help yourself. Start by breaking the cycle of ongoing pain with my REST protocol.

REST PROTOCOL

- **R**educe your morning pain as much as possible.
- **E**valuate and modify or eliminate the activity that makes your pain worse.
- **S**hoes that are appropriate for all activity and help— not hurt—you.
- **T**ry off-the-shelf solutions that reduce compensations and the likelihood for secondary injury.

The **R** part of **REST** is to reduce your morning pain (or pain after rest) as much as possible. You do this in two ways: with simple and effective targeted stretches as soon as you wake up, *before standing up*, and by wearing your running shoes to take your first steps in the morning.

The **E** part of **REST** is evaluate. I want you to look at your daily activities and modify or eliminate the ones that make your pain worse. At the same time, I want you to stay active through plantar fasciitis. Until you read chapter 7, cut out planks, lunges, running, and anything else that extends your toes back during activity.

The **S** part of **REST** is shoes. Proper footwear plays a crucial role in treating plantar fasciitis. Make sure you're wearing your running shoes as much as possible, even around the house and especially *first thing in the morning*.

The **T** part of **REST** is try off-the-shelf solutions. Your local pharmacy is a great source of inexpensive solutions for foot pain, such as heel cups and padded inserts for your shoes. These devices are put into your shoe as a way to help you walk more comfortably so you don't hurt yourself more.

CHAPTER 6

TIMING

R ecovery can take anywhere from six weeks to three years. The sooner you get treatment, the sooner you will recover, but some people just take longer than others, even with prompt treatment. In my experience, the majority of people will take between six weeks to a year to heal. It's only the worst cases, when things really go badly or become resistant to treatment, that result in a person being in pain for three years. In very rare cases, the pain remains chronic.

We all recover at different rates and different times, and lots of factors play into recovery. Some modifiable factors will speed your recovery, however.

GET TREATED EARLY

First, get on the pain early. If you get your heel pain diagnosed and begin treatment as soon as you can, you have a better chance of getting better faster (Michelsoson et al. 2005). If you let it go for months, as many of my patients do, you slow down your recovery. We know from the scientific literature that if you get control of your pain within seven months of the first symptoms, you're many times more likely to get better than if you're in pain longer than seven months.

MODIFY YOUR WORKING CONDITIONS

Look into modifying your working conditions. If you work too much of the time on hard floors, it's going to take you longer to get better. Those hard surfaces are a risk factor to getting plantar fasciitis to begin with. If you can't change that part of your job, your healing will be much slower. Based on your pain level and your ability to be productive and active at work, ask your supervisor or the HR department if you can go on light or modified duty. (See chapter 19 for an explanation of your right to have your request honored.)

I would want you to take it easy and stay off hard surfaces even if you're wearing orthotics. The orthotics will help you do your job with less pain, but they're not magic, and you will still have pain if you have to walk on a hard surface all day.

EAT BETTER AND LOSE WEIGHT

Take a good look at your nutrition. Eating "properly" is important for your recovery. That means good quality, nutrient-dense foods, not empty calories from soft drinks, junk food, and highly processed foods. You can get 2,000 calories from a huge burger, or you can get 2,000 calories from high-quality protein, fats, and low-glycemic carbohydrates, including lots of colorful vegetables.

The burger won't give your body the nutritional building blocks it needs to heal.

I consider weight loss to be part of looking at your nutrition. Excess weight is a risk factor in itself for PF (Irving et al. 2006). Every time you take a step, 1.25 times your body weight goes through your foot. If you're managing to take the recommended ten thousand steps a day for good fitness, even an extra five or ten pounds can add up fast in terms of additional load on your foot. Being heavier than that just adds to the load and makes the risk even greater. If you're a runner or active in some other way (tennis, soccer, etc.), up to three times your body weight goes through your foot with every stride. Over the course of a 10K race, that's thousands and thousands of pounds putting extra strain on your plantar fascia.

I'm not qualified to tell you how to lose weight. That's as individual as treating PF. (Remember what I said about being terrified about fitting one lone solution to everyone's problems.) Instead, I recommend working with a professional who can design a workable program for you. I worked online with an expert coach at Precision Nutrition (precisionnutrition.com) and lost forty-five pounds. They will teach you solid nutritional habits are the key to success.

GET GOOD SLEEP

Good sleep is important for healing, because our bodies recover from injury when we sleep. It's the body's time to make repairs. Poor sleep quality and duration are definitely going to prevent you from healing to your best ability. Today it's easier to learn more about your sleep quality than ever before. You don't have to just wake up and realize you don't feel rested. Inexpensive wearable devices can now tell you what your sleep duration was and what its quality was. The devices record how much you move during your sleep and can tell you how much deep sleep you got. This is helpful, because you do the most recovery and healing during deep sleep. If you know you don't sleep well, or if you feel terrible in the morning, even though you slept for eight hours, it may be time to talk to your doctor. Something else might be going on. You might be stressed out, have sleep apnea, or maybe you have another medical condition. Or you could be overcaffeinated, like me!

You can do some simple things to improve the quality of your sleep.

* Limit your exposure to the blue light of TVs, computer screens, smartphones, and tablets. Studies have shown that blue light in the evening can cause insomnia, plus blue light is bad for your retinas. Avoid these devices for two hours before bedtime.
* Instead of watching TV or playing a video game, try reading, talking with your significant other, playing with your dog— anything that's enjoyable and relaxing before you go to sleep.
* Make the bedroom as dark as possible. Even after you close the blinds or curtains, the typical bedroom today is full of light-emitting devices such as the clock, the cable box, and the phone. Cover all of those little lights with electrical tape or put the device in a drawer.
* Keep the bedroom on the cool side. Research suggest that 18° C (65° F) is the ideal temperature.
* Avoid physical activity two hours before calling it a night. If you like to work out in the evening, just do it earlier.

RECOVERY

You'll know you've achieved a full recovery when you no longer have any pain in your foot. There's no pain when you get out of bed, no pain after rest, and no pain after activity. If you get to that point and you start having pain again a couple of months later, it could be that you just weren't fully recovered or you went back to things too quickly.

I tell a lot of my people they need to take three months off from their weight-bearing activity. They do, and then they're so excited about feeling better that they go from ten-minute walks with the dog to a two-hour hike. That's almost guaranteed to bring the pain back. Your return to your usual activity level should be gradual. On the other hand, a small amount of residual pain for several months after you have basically recovered isn't unusual. It's probably because you have a bit of nerve irritation. Nerves heal very slowly.

Unfortunately, some professionals stick to the outdated advice that nothing really helps PF except staying off your feet. If you do that for nine months to a year, the PF will go away on its own. Unfortunately, the prevailing wisdom of today is easily ten years behind the best and most current treatment ideas. Would you tell someone with any other sort of injury to just not do anything for nine months? I know from clinical experience that we can get you better faster without asking you to be inactive for nine months or longer.

PREVENTION

Plantar fasciitis is easier to prevent than heal. You can't fix things like high arches, but you can minimize your risk factors by trying to keep your weight down, keeping your flexibility and your range of motion up, and mitigating other risk factors such as hard surfaces for long periods of time and training errors. The other important thing you can do to prevent PF is keep your feet as strong as possible. If the supporting musculature of your foot and ankle is strong, PF is less likely. I'll be discussing pre-vention and the problem of recurrence in more detail in chapter 20. Once you've had PF, you're more susceptible to getting it again, so it's important to stay aware and keep your feet strong.

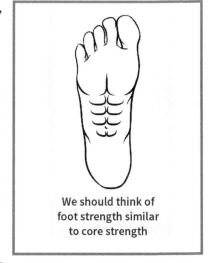

We should think of foot strength similar to core strength

LOW-COST SOLUTIONS

Plantar fasciitis can be treated with some very helpful, noninvasive, low-cost solutions. I'll go into all of them in later chapters. For now, let's just list them:

- Stretches
- Changing your activity
- Changing your footwear
- Being more mindful of your gait and avoiding compensating
- Trying low-cost, off-the-shelf orthotics

REST TO BREAK THE PAIN CYCLE

Introduction

Plantar fasciitis is an injury of half-healing and retearing. The reason people come to me after they've been sore for months is that they don't understand that their first ten steps are the most important ten steps of their day. That's when you're doing the most damage for the rest of the day. The treatment for PF isn't to do nothing—that's not an answer. Instead, break the cycle of re-injury and ongoing pain with my REST protocol.

REST Protocol

- **R**educe your morning pain as much as possible.
- **E**valuate and modify or eliminate the activity that makes your pain worse.
- **S**hoes that are appropriate for all activity and help—not hurt—you.
- **T**ry off-the-shelf solutions that reduce compensations and the likelihood for secondary injury.

The **R** part of **REST** is to *reduce* your pain after rest as much as possible. You do this in two ways: with simple and effective targeted stretches as soon as you wake up and by wearing your shoes first thing in the morning. The goal of this first phase of treatment is for you to be able to get up and have less pain with your first ten steps. You won't be cured overnight, but we're definitely going to make tomorrow morning a better morning.

The **E** part of **REST** is *evaluate*. I want you to look at your daily activities and modify or eliminate the ones that make your pain worse. At the same time, you want to stay active through plantar fasciitis. In later chapters, I'll explain how you can change things around so that you're not making your pain worse while you continue to be active. You'll avoid weight gain and loss of fitness.

The **S** part of **REST** is *shoes*. I'll explain the crucial role footwear plays in treating plantar fasciitis in chapter 10.

The **T** part of **REST** is *try* off-the-shelf solutions. Your local pharmacy is a great source of inexpensive solutions for foot pain, such as heel cups and padded inserts for your shoes. These devices are put into your shoe as a way to help you walk more comfortably so you don't hurt yourself more. They help reduce the likelihood of a secondary injury.

These steps are meant to be done all together as a group of treatments for a minimum of six weeks.

CHAPTER 7

REDUCE YOUR MORNING PAIN AS MUCH AS POSSIBLE

Pain is your body's way of saying, this is too much. It's a warning signal, it's a gift we're given that we don't pay attention to.
—Irene S. Davis, PhD

The R in REST stands for reduce. You can reduce your morning pain and pain after rest significantly with some simple yet effective targeted foot stretches done first thing in the morning before you even get out of bed. The stretching exercises help reduce your pain by breaking up the cycle of half-healing and retearing. This is the most important part of the REST protocol.

The stretches work to break up that cycle by warming up the range of motion in your foot before you put weight on it. The stretches also break down the scar tissue, getting your foot ready to go so that you don't retear and have as much morning pain with your first ten steps. You'll still have morning pain, but if you do these stretches every single morning, your pain will gradually reduce.

STRETCHING BASICS

When we look at the science on what kind of stretching to do for plantar fasciitis, two different protocols stand out. There's the generic approach, which focused on stretching the calf muscles as you stand against a wall. Then there's the more targeted approach of doing tissue-specific stretching of your plantar fascia. The research shows that the targeted approach is more effective than the generic approach (DiGiovanni et al. 2003). The targeted approach also doesn't require you to get out of bed and take your first ten steps in order to reach a wall to do calf stretches. The specific stretches I recommend for PF are done *before you put weight on your foot in the morning*. These stretches set your foot up for the best-case scenario before you put a load on your plantar fascia. You do them when you first wake up, sitting on the edge of your bed. You only have to stretch the affected foot. To see the best way to do the stretches, visit **thepfplan.com/videos**. I walk you through all the exercises in the video.

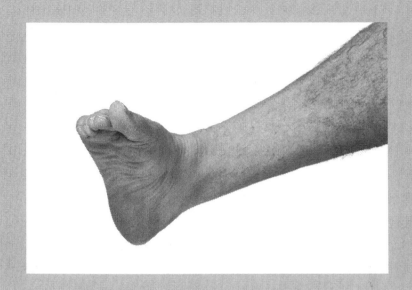

Ankle Rotation

This exercise helps improve the range of motion in your ankle. Better range of motion means less strain on the plantar fascia. This stretch will take your foot and ankle through all the different ranges of motion:

- Sit on the edge of your bed with your leg outstretched and knee straight.
- Make slow, controlled circles with your foot, as if you were "writing" the alphabet with your foot.
- "Write" the alphabet once.

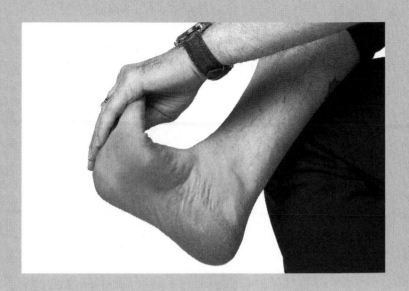

Toe Extensions

This stretch lengthens the plantar fascia:

- Sit on the edge of your bed.
- Place the affected foot across the opposite knee.
- Cup your heel with one hand and grasp your toes with the other.
- Pull your toes and ankle toward your shin until you feel the stretch in your arch. Never pull past the point of pain.
- Hold the stretch for 10 to 15 seconds; do the stretch five times.

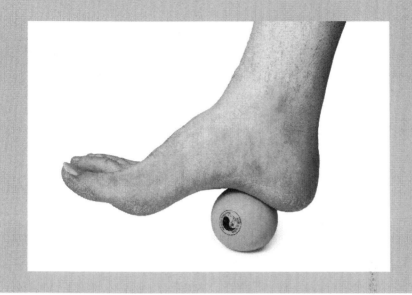

Arch Massage

This stretch uses a tennis ball to massage the arch of your foot. It can be mildly uncomfortable; the pain should improve over time. Some people like to use a massage ball or roller instead:

- Sit on the edge of the bed with your feet flat on the floor.
- Place a tennis ball under the arch of the affected foot.
- Roll your foot over the ball while pushing down on it, starting at the heel and moving to the ball of your foot.
- Keep it up for one minute.

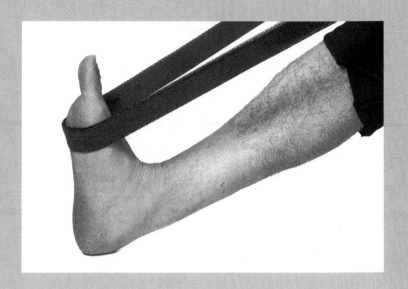

Seated Calf Stretch

This exercise stretches out tight calf and hamstring muscles:

- Sit on the edge of the bed with the affected leg outstretched.
- Hook a belt or towel around your toes and use it to pull your foot toward you while keeping the knee straight.
- Hold for 30 seconds.
- To help avoid gait imbalance, do this stretch for both legs. If you feel discomfort in the knee, back off on pulling your foot back too much.

EXTRA STRETCHING

Aside from doing your stretches faithfully every morning before you get out of bed, I recommend doing them whenever you've been seated for longer than twenty minutes, say at your desk or in the car. Depending on where you are, you may not be able to do all four stretches, but do as many as you can as often as you can after you've been sitting for a while. I suggest keeping a tennis ball in a desk drawer so you can kick off your shoes and give yourself a foot massage.

PUT YOUR SHOES ON

Once you've finished your morning stretches, put on your running shoes before you take a step. **Do not walk barefoot.** The stretches have broken down the scar tissue, warmed up the range of motion, and gotten everything ready to go. Now we want to protect and cushion the foot by wearing shoes. By shoes, I mean running shoes that fit well, not slippers.

DO YOU NEED PHYSICAL THERAPY?

Physical therapy can be helpful for treating PF. I'm not a physical therapist, so I can't say if it would be right for you or not. Fortunately, I know an awesome physical therapist who can answer those questions. I've asked Greg Alcock, MSc(PT), BA Hons(PE), FCAMPT, physiotherapy clinical and research coordinator at the Fowler Kennedy Clinic in London, Ontario, for his expert thoughts. Here's what he says:

> Not all cases of plantar fasciitis are created equal. Each case has its own unique set of contributing factors. This can make PF difficult to understand as a patient, to treat as a medical

*professional, and to study as researchers. This is also why
there isn't a conclusive treatment approach that solves all
cases. The information below is meant to be a starting point
for consideration. It's in no way exhaustive in covering
all the available aspects of this complex but common
clinical problem.*

*First, seek information. The more information you have, the
better for understanding your condition—but make sure it's good
information. Surfing the Internet, asking the local running group,
or getting cornered by Aunt Jean at the family summer picnic
telling you that "cousin Larry has the exact same problem…" is
often well intentioned, but it doesn't make your pain go away.
Seek advice from a professional.*

The basic checklist for choosing a good physical therapist includes
the following:

- The therapist should qualify as a physical therapist under
  Canadian or your location's regulations.
- At your first visit, your therapist should perform a thorough
  subjective history, physical, and biomechanical exam. The
  therapist is looking for any contributing factors from your lumbar
  spine down to your foot—you want to make sure you truly have
  plantar fasciitis!
- The therapist should explain your condition in terms of
  modifiable and non-modifiable risk factors and how the
  treatment plan is going to address these issues. This may include
  a variety of approaches, from exercise, manual therapy, and
  various modalities to referral to other health-care professionals.

- The therapist should be familiar with the published clinical practice guidelines relating to PF. These are helpful for developing a customized treatment plan that considers the available evidence for all potential options, from splinting to platelet rich plasma (PRP) injections.

The treatment approach your PT recommends may be less important than the results. Treatments may vary, but results need to be evaluated. Essential questions you should ask yourself as treatment goes on are as follows:

- Am I getting better?
- Am I able to do more of the things that I was limited in doing because of my symptoms?
- Is this happening in a reasonable amount of time?

Your therapist should help you determine this using a validated outcome measure. There are many of these—they're usually simple pen and paper questionnaires.

If the physical therapy hasn't changed your symptoms in a meaningful way in a reasonable amount of time, your therapist should help you interpret this and revisit the treatment approach you have developed together.

Taping can be clinically valuable for evaluating and treating plantar fasciitis in some, although not all, cases. Taping is often used to modify a contributing factor identified in the assessment portion of the exam. The area is taped to see if it makes your symptoms worse, better, or the same. Taping can assist in clinically reasoning through the approach to your treatment progression. It isn't always necessary, but if it's needed, make sure it's done correctly. The only thing worse than no tape job is a poor tape job— you don't want to have plantar fasciitis and blisters! Taping your own foot is difficult based on geometry and anatomy. It's like cutting your own hair. Just because you can doesn't mean you should.

Treating plantar fasciitis requires a comprehensive approach from therapist and patient. It is unrealistic to hope that, in isolation, a periodic visit to the physical therapy clinic will "fix" your condition. The real value is developing and evaluating a good treatment plan with your therapist that is specific to your needs. This involves some commitment. The patient has to agree to follow the treatment plan on a daily basis outside the clinic between visits: exercises, stretching, activity modification, a change in footwear, and other responsibilities.

CHAPTER 8

EVALUATE YOUR ACTIVITY

The next step in the REST protocol is E: Evaluate your activity and modify or eliminate anything that makes your pain worse. The goal is always to keep you as active as you usually are. In general, it's important to stay active to help control your weight. I want you to avoid gaining weight because you're less active. But even more importantly, the reason to stay active through your plantar fasciitis is to avoid reducing your health-related quality of life. Studies have shown that people who have chronic heel pain, specifically chronic plantar fasciitis, score lower on health-related quality of life measures than people who don't. A 2016 study in the journal *Foot & Ankle International* suggested that people who have chronic heel pain suffer greater depression, anxiety, and stress (Cotchett et al. 2016). Your ability to participate in your usual activities of daily living, have a social life, go to work, and do things you enjoy all go down when you have chronic foot pain. A decrease in health-related quality of life can lead, at its worst, to feeling very stressed or even depressed. I have a client, a young woman who suffers from depression. She copes with it very well by running. She says that seeing me isn't about getting her orthotics for her foot pain, it's about her quality of life. I want all my patients to have the best possible quality of life while they cope with plantar fasciitis.

Another really big reason for staying active is to manage any other disorders you may have, such as lower back pain, and to avoid getting any new disorders. Someone with prediabetes who gets much less active may tip over into diabetes, for instance. Staying physically active also keeps your blood flowing. The plantar fascia is poorly vascularized. The more active you are, the more you maximize the blood flow to the area. Better blood flow brings oxygen and nutrition, as well as the body's natural anti-inflammatory chemicals, to the area and carries away wastes.

THE RULES

I have two rules for staying active during injury.

Number 1: Don't do anything that makes it worse during or after.
Number 2: See rule Number 1.

Don't make it worse. That's not always as simple as it sounds. The problem with plantar fasciitis is that often people will be able to stay active and not have any pain once they get past their first morning steps. If you're functioning with a low baseline level of pain, you can go running; you can play soccer; you can play tennis. It's only after you sit down at the end of these activities and then go to get back up again, or when you get up the next morning, that you feel the damage. That's when you're in more pain, not when you were being active the day before. If your plantar fasciitis is bad enough that it's painful while you're doing your activity, you simply have to cut that activity out completely until you recover.

Typically, I tell people that pain shouldn't be increased during or after activity. If you have more pain during, stop. If you have more pain after, then you want to reduce what you did by 15 to 20 percent at first. Try the activity again to see if the pain afterward is better. If it isn't, keep cutting it back, possibly to the point where you just don't do it for now. You might find that you can still play a round of golf, but maybe it means walking for nine holes and carting for the back nine instead of walking the full eighteen, or carting for the full course.

ACTIVITIES TO AVOID

The activities to avoid are things that put your toes in an extended position. Your plantar fascia tightens up when your toes are extended back to make your foot a more rigid lever to help propel you forward. Examples would be crouching down and putting your weight on the balls of your feet and/or the toes. That is bad for your plantar fascia. Similarly, gardening in a kneeling position, with your toes cranked back behind you or digging into the ground, isn't a good idea. Any sort of exercise activity that makes you dig in your toes or push off of them is likely to be painful and even cause more damage. Exercises like planks, lunges, calf raises, seated or standing sled pushes, and certain yoga poses all put you in a bad dynamic position. You want to avoid or modify these activities.

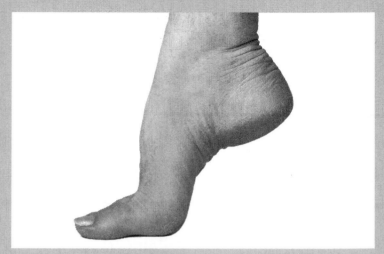

Try to reduce placing your foot in this position as much as possible.

I want you to stay active, so I always recommend trying to modify an exercise instead of eliminating it. For example, you will probably want to modify planks, because they put your toes in a bad position. Instead of a regular plank, you can do a modified version. Put a foam roller underneath the front part of your ankle to help you stay in the basic plank position without extending back your toes. Instead of a lunge, do a step up. Instead of going into a crouching position where you're extending your toes back, just keep your feet flat, or kneel and put your feet straight out behind you. There's no way around calf raises. Just stop doing them for now, unless you're told by a physiotherapist that they could be of benefit. Sled pushing puts all your weight on the balls of your feet. You want to just take that one out for now.

Even though yoga is recommended as a way to stretch and become more flexible, some yoga poses are actually really bad for plantar fasciitis. Any yoga pose that has you go up on your toes should be avoided. That includes poses such as downward dog and various toe stands. Fortunately, plenty of yoga poses don't involve the toes—a good yoga instructor can help you find poses you can do comfortably. You'll also want to stay away from step aerobics class, Zumba, and any strenuous dance class. Anything that involves dynamic jumping, which is forefoot intensive, should be avoided. Instead, try replacing it with the elliptical machine or another form of low-impact cardio.

Running, jogging, weight-bearing activity, and explosive weight-bearing activity (plyometrics) should all be avoided or modified. Degenerative changes to the plantar fascia can happen if you've had the problem for a long time, or if it has become chronic. The more degenerated your plantar fascia becomes, the stiffer and more inelastic it is. At this stage, the risk of rupture is greater, so it's particularly important to avoid highly explosive dynamic activity. If you want to continue to cross-train, do things that are a little bit less explosive, with less pounding on your heel.

Bike riding is fine if you have plantar fasciitis. Also fine are swimming, handcycles, and basic body weight circuit training. Check out low-impact cardio alternates, such as a rowing machine; the Octane Zero Runner, which mimics the action of running without any impact on your feet; or the Octane Lateral X Elliptical. Anything else you enjoy and that doesn't make your feet hurt during or after is also fine. I encourage you to explore new activities while you heal.

ALTERNATIVE EXERCISES

While you're healing from plantar fasciitis, you need to modify your activity. Running, jogging, long fast walks, dancing, aerobics class, and any other activity that puts stress and strain on your foot should be avoided for now. At the same time, it's important to stay active and to keep as fit as you can. To help you learn some alternative exercises that won't hurt your foot, I asked personal trainer April Crake, I.S.S.A. Cert., BSc (KIN), for some variations on standard exercises. For each of these exercises, start with one set. When that becomes easy and you feel ready to progress, add up to three sets.

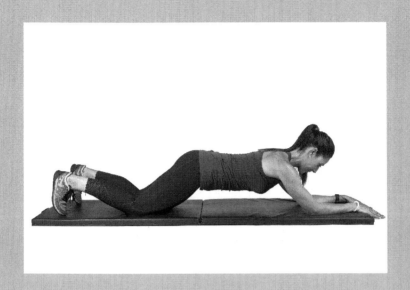

Eight-Point Plank (Plank Alternative)

- Lie on your stomach with your feet flexed, knees touching, and elbows a few inches in front of your shoulders.
- Pull your shoulders away from your ears; gently squeeze the knees and elbows toward the centerline of your body.
- Press knees, toes, and elbows into the mat as you lift your hips up to the height of the shoulders.
- Tighten your core and maintain a long, neutral spine.
- Pull the elbows and knees toward each other (as though you're trying to bring the top and bottom of your mat together), and hold the plank for 20 to 30 seconds.

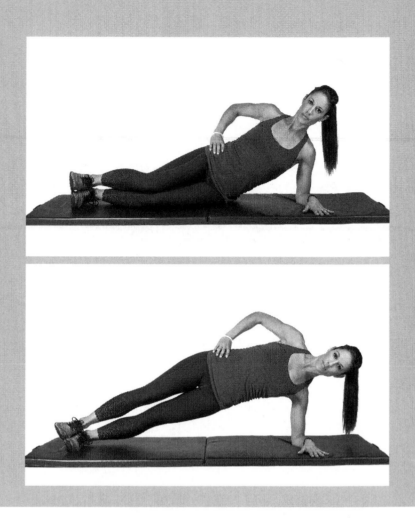

Kneeling Side Plank (Plank Alternative)

- Bend your legs at the knee at a right angle and keep your thighs and torso in line.
- Your forearm, elbow, knee, and lower leg are your points of contact with the ground.

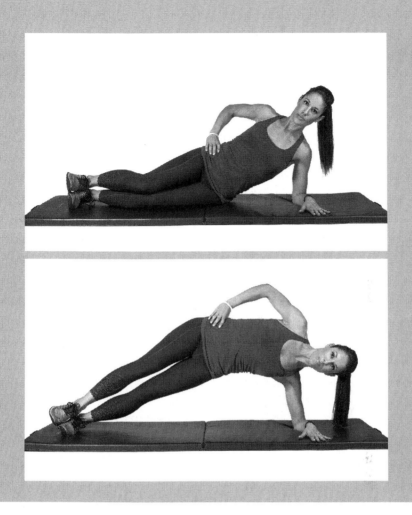

Side Plank with Hip Raise (Plank Alternative)

- Start on your side, with legs stacked and feet flexed, resting one forearm on the floor.
- Place opposite hand on hip (for balance). Lift into side plank.
- Hold for 2 counts.
- Raise and lower hips 10 to 12 times. Switch sides. Repeat.

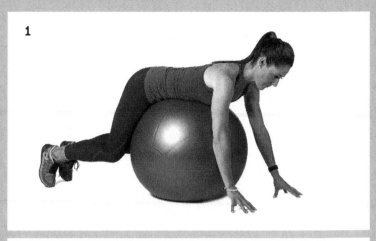

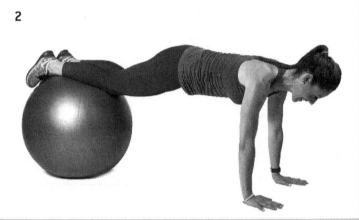

Exercise Ball Knee Tucks (Plank Alternative)

- Kneel in front of an exercise ball and place your hands about shoulder-width apart on the floor.
- Extend your legs one at a time behind you to rest on top of the ball.
- Lift your hips so they are in line with your heels and head.

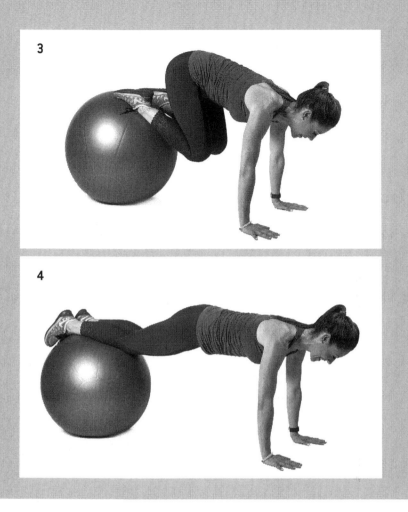

- Drive your knees toward your chest and then extend them back out until you form a solid plank position.
- Repeat 10 to 20 times.

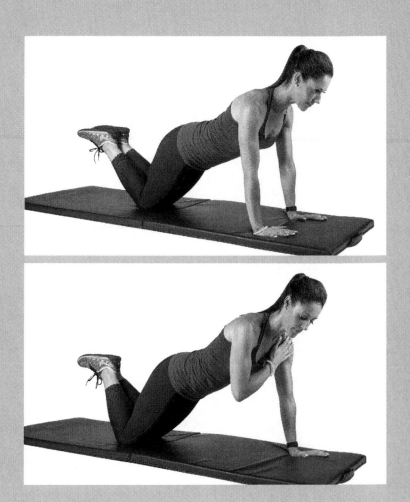

Plank Shoulder Taps (Plank Alternative)

- Get into a push-up position with your hands shoulder-width apart on the floor and your shins resting on top of the exercise ball.
- Keep your hips square to the floor while you lift your right hand and tap your left shoulder.
- Return to start and repeat with the other arm.
- Continue alternating for a total of 20 reps.

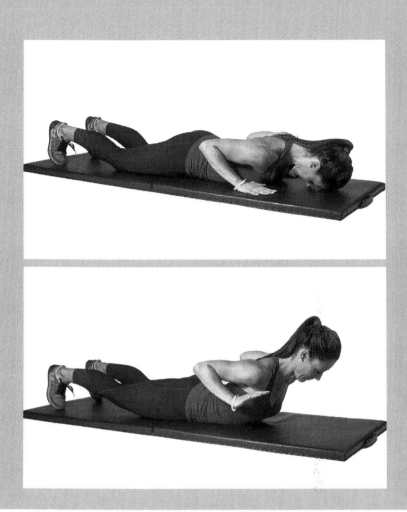

Adductor-Assisted Back Extension (Plank Alternative)

- Lie on your stomach. Flex your feet and zip your legs together, keeping just a slight bend at the knees.
- Press your hips and knees into the ground and lift your elbows up until the hands "float" above the ground. Pull your shoulders down toward your glutes while lifting your chest off the ground. Keep your neck long.
- Hold for 20 to 30 seconds.

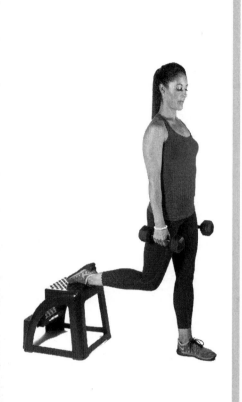
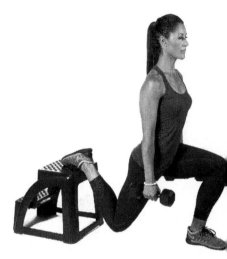

Bulgarian Split Squats (Lunge Alternative)

- Stand lunge-length in front of a bench.
- Hold dumbbells in each hand and rest the top of your left foot on the bench behind you.
- Lower your body until your rear knee nearly touches the floor and your front thigh is parallel to the floor.
- 4. Do 10 to 15 reps on one leg and then switch to the other leg.

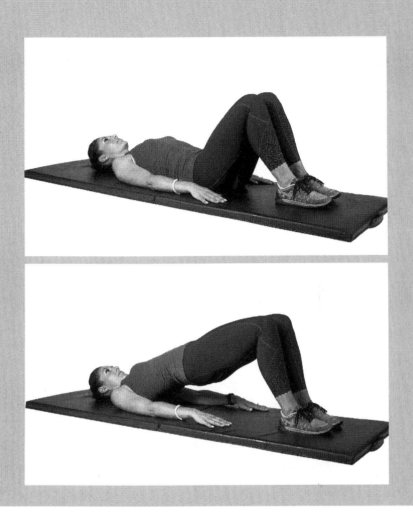

Bodyweight Hip Raises (Lunge Alternative)

- Lie on your back, lift your glutes and hips up, and squeeze your glutes. Pause for 1 second and then lower.
- To make it more challenging, put your feet on a step or exercise ball.

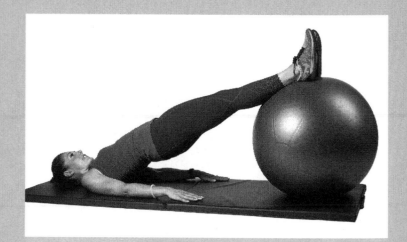

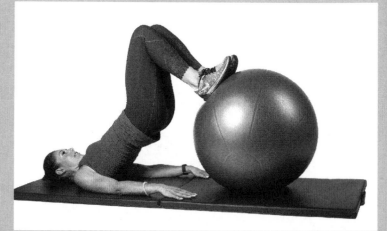

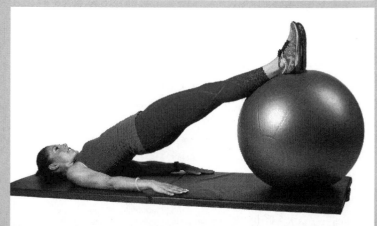

Exercise Ball Glute Raise and Hamstring Curl
(Advanced Lunge Alternative)

- Lie face up on the floor, arms out to the sides, and lower legs on the exercise ball.
- Push your hips up until your body forms a straight line from shoulders to knees.
- Pull your heels toward you and roll the ball as close as possible to your butt.
- Pause and then roll the ball back until your body is in a straight line again—that's 1 rep.
- Do 10 to 15 reps.

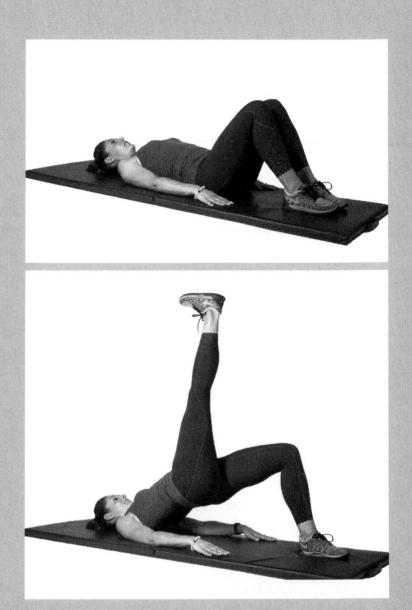

Single-Leg Hip Raise (Lunge Alternative)

- Lie face up on the floor with your left knee bent and right leg straight. Your right leg should be in line with your left thigh.
- Make your stomach as tight as possible and hold it.
- Squeeze your glutes and raise your hips until your body forms a straight line from your shoulders to your knees. Your torso and hips should move as one unit. Your left leg should stay elevated the entire time.
- Pause for 2 seconds, continuing to keep your abs tight and squeeze your glutes.
- Lower back to the starting position.
- Do 8 to 10 reps.

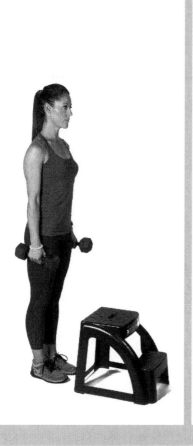
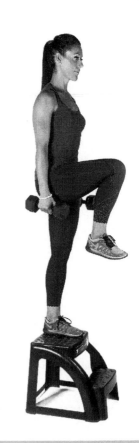

Step-Ups with Knee Raise (Lunge Alternative)

- Place a 12- to 24-inch step in front of you. Step up with your left foot, bringing your right leg forward and up and bending your knee until your thigh is parallel to the floor.
- Lower your right leg back to start and then repeat with right foot and left leg. That's 1 rep.
- Do 10 reps.

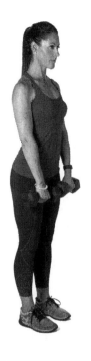
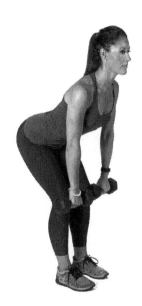

Dumbbell Straight-Leg Deadlift (Lunge Alternative)

- Hold 5- to 8-pound dumbbells in front of your thighs. Stand with feet hip-width apart and knees slightly bent.
- Bend at your hips to lower your torso until it's almost parallel to the floor, keeping the weights close to your body.
- Return to standing, keeping the weights close to your body.
- Do 8 to 10 reps.

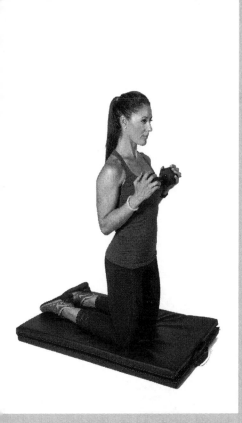 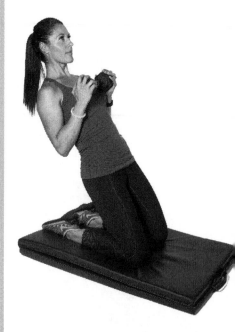

The Matrix (Lunge Alternative)

- Hold a 5- to 10-pound medicine ball, dumbbell, or kettlebell and kneel on the floor with your knees hip-width apart. Lengthen your spine and press the weight against your abs.
- Slowly lean back as far as possible, keeping your knees planted.
- Hold the reclined position for 3 seconds and then use your core to slowly come up to the starting position. That's 1 rep.
- Start slow, and go to 10 reps.

CHAPTER 9

SHOES THAT HELP

Give a girl the right shoes, and she can conquer the world.

—Marilyn Monroe

T he S in REST stands for shoes. To recover from plantar fasciitis, you need shoes that are appropriate for your activity and that will help, not hurt, you.

PICKING FOOTWEAR BASED ON FOOT TYPE

Before you choose footwear to improve plantar fasciitis, you need to know what kind of foot you have. In particular, you want to know what kind of arch you have. In a study published in 2012 entitled "Runner's Knowledge of Their Foot Type: Do They Really Know?" the researchers reported that of the ninety-two runners they surveyed, less than half (49 percent) were able to correctly identify their foot type (Hohmann et al. 2012). The implication of this research may suggest that due to runners' seemly poor knowledge of their own foot type, there may be a greater chance they will pick the wrong shoe and perhaps be at a greater risk of injury.

Until recently, research on military and female runner populations have suggested that the influence of matching one's foot type to a particular style of shoe was not particularly effective. In 2016, a study in the *British Journal of Sports Medicine* suggested that injury risk was lower among lower-arched runners who wore motion-control shoes (Malisoux et al. 2016). This was a well-designed trial where both the runners and the researchers were blind to who was running in which shoes. The findings of this paper were in contrast to research published in the same journal by Ryan et al. in 2011, which suggested that in female runners, in-shoe, motion-control features might actually be causing pain in some instances (Ryan et al. 2011). Based on the strengths of the Malisoux paper, some of the weaknesses of past research, and testing the theory with patients over time, I believe there is merit in suggesting footwear to match foot types both to try and reduce injury rates and to reduce the likelihood of injury from using a shoe opposite to your individual biomechanics.

WHAT KIND OF ARCH DO YOU HAVE?

To help arm you with better knowledge of your foot type, you can do a very simple test at home called the wet foot test or the paper test. This test is credited to Colonel R. I. Harris and Major T. Beath, who used the test on Canadian soldiers to evaluate issues related to their feet (Knapik et al. 2014). Open out a brown paper bag or lay down some newspaper on the floor; tape the paper to the floor. Remove your shoes and socks and lightly wet the bottoms of your

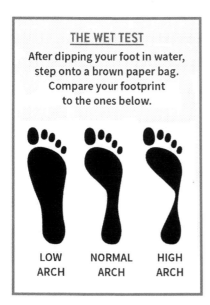

THE WET TEST

After dipping your foot in water, step onto a brown paper bag. Compare your footprint to the ones below.

LOW ARCH   NORMAL ARCH   HIGH ARCH

feet. Walk across the paper. You'll leave a wet footprint. If you compare the outline to the ones in the diagram, you can see if you have a high, medium, or low arch.

It's possible that if you have a low arch and you do get plantar fasciitis, you're going to be slow to heal. In theory, that's because your low arch puts excess strain on the soft tissues in your plantar fascia. There's no evidence, however, that having a low arch will cause PF. In fact, having a high arch, with less flexibility, puts you more at risk.

Based on what you now know about your arch, you can choose the right type of athletic shoe for your foot. To be more precise, you can avoid buying the wrong type of shoe. Running shoe technology has advanced quite a bit over the years, but runners still get injured in their shoes. The evidence shows that getting a shoe that's wrong for your foot type may cause pain. Don't get too carried away with the results of the wet foot test, though. Static measures of feet may not tell the entire story. What happens dynamically can also affect shoe selection, and that's why I advocate seeing a professional who can take them both into account.

Let's say you have a really high arch and spend more time on the outside of your foot when you run. If you get a shoe that's meant to push you that way, then you might overcorrect yourself and wind up with a new injury. If someone who's a supinator—the foot rolls away from the midline of the body with each stride—gets into an anti-pronator shoe, that would be the opposite shoe for their foot type. Pronators roll their feet toward the midline. When a supinator wears an anti-pronation shoe, they may get pain on the outside of their ankle or their foot, because the shoe is exaggerating what their foot wants to do. We want a shoe to either counteract what your foot wants to do or complement it; that will remove some of the strain on the soft tissues.

If you have a low-arched foot, you typically have a lot of mobility in your feet, and you can absorb shock very well. Your foot type is adaptable to changing direction. If you have a really high-arched foot, typically your foot is very rigid. It doesn't absorb shock very well, and you wind up with more shock-related injuries. If you have a normal foot, then your foot doesn't pronate a lot; it doesn't supinate a lot. It just moves a little bit in each direction, which is fine.

Running magazines are full of articles about how pronation is bad for you. That's not really the case. It's the normal movement for most people who have normal to low-arched feet, because it helps to reduce load when you walk or run. In some cases, prona-tion puts more strain on your foot, but having a super-low-arched foot doesn't predict a problem. I have some patients whose feet are so flat their full arch touches the ground, but they are Iron-man triathletes and are pain free. My thinking for people with flat feet isn't give them orthotics as a first-line treatment, it's get them into the right footwear.

GETTING THE RIGHT FIT

Now that you understand what foot type you have, you want to find a shoe that fits your individual biomechanics. You want the right shoe for the activity. You want the overall size to be right; you want the heel-to-toe fit to be right, and you want the right width. If the shoe doesn't fit well in any one of those areas, it's not right for you. You may injure yourself or end up with a sore foot.

Here's what to look for in a good fit:

- **Heel to toe.** The longest toe should be accommodated, with approximately 7 mm, or about a pinky finger's width, between the longest toe and the end of the shoe.
- **Heel to ball (arch length).** This aspect of fit is often overlooked, but it's extremely important. Make sure that the widest part of your foot lines up with the widest part of the shoe (the "flex point").
- **Heel fit.** The heel counters (the hard part that holds the heel) of shoes are made in different widths and back curves. If your heel slips even though you have laced the shoe properly, try an alternate style.
- **Width.** This can be subjective to your overall comfort. Too narrow and you toes will go numb. Too wide and the foot will not be adequately secure.
- **Socks.** When fitting shoes, be sure to wear the socks you will be using with them. Dress, work, and athletic socks can all be different thicknesses and may result in a difference in fit.

When buying shoes, I recommend doing it toward the end of the day, when your feet are a bit swollen from the day's activity. You'll get a better fit that way.

HEEL HEIGHT

The height of the heel—the offset between your heel and your forefoot—in activity shoes can range anywhere from a zero drop to 12 mm. Shoe manufacturers have now started offering lower heel heights so that you strike less on your heel and more on the middle of your foot. If you have plantar fasciitis, you actually want to elevate your heel a bit to decrease the pull from your Achilles tendon and take some of the pressure off your heel. I typically recommend a heel height between 10 and 12 mm to keep your heel elevated a bit. Lower heel heights are more like walking barefoot, which for PF isn't a good thing. Here's where things go crazy. You want to say, "But dude, I *love* my barefoot shoes." That's OK—keep wearing them. By now, I think you get the point that we're all different, and what works for one won't work for all. I've seen some cases where people have improved with the use of barefoot shoes. But I've also seen cases where people have gotten stress fractures from barefoot shoes. There is research to support both sides of the argument, and one hasn't outweighed the other, yet. Personally and professionally, I don't advocate wearing barefoot shoes if you have PF.

GETTING THE RIGHT CATEGORY

When you go to the shoe store, use your knowledge of your arch type to figure out what shoe category you fit into. You'll probably fall into one of four categories: cushioning, stable neutral, stability, or motion control.

- Cushioning shoes offer ample cushioning and a little bit of support. This is appropriate for someone who has a normal foot type to a higher-arched foot and is a bit of a supinator. The shoe will give you a lot of cushioning but not a lot of support.

- Stable neutral shoes still have lots of cushioning, but provide a bit more support for the inside part of your foot. If you have a normal- to low-arched foot, you might do well in a stable neutral shoe.
- Stability shoes have a moderate amount of stability and a little bit of cushioning. Stability shoes usually have more support on the inside part of the shoe. The material itself is usually 10 to 15 percent stiffer on the inside part of the shoe. It's meant to resist pronation.
- Motion-control shoes have firm support on both the inside and the outside of the shoe. They're typically completely filled in on the bottom. These are stiffest shoes you can get, which also means they're among the heaviest shoes you can get. These shoes can give you so much support that you overcorrect your foot, which can lead to a new and different injury. Most people don't need motion-control shoes. If you think you do, talk to a foot specialist or go to a specialty shoe store first.

A note on minimalist shoes. These became very popular when barefoot running became a craze. Now that the benefits of barefoot running have become more controversial, these shoes are less popular. They don't have much cushioning. They have very thin midsoles, so you're closer to the ground overall. Minimalist shoes are very, very flexible, so if you're a pronator, the shoe will allow you to continue to pronate. If you're a real supinator, it's going to allow you to continue to supinate. The shoe is really just meant to be a layer between your foot and the ground to provide some protection from the elements and the running surface.

If you're shopping at a large athletics store with a big wall of shoes, the salespeople may be able to help you narrow down the choices, but it can be hit or miss. I advocate for the smaller specialty store, where the salespeople have more expertise.

Want to test them yourself? To see if a shoe falls in the category of cushioning or stability, do three tests. First, pick it up by the heel and toe and try to wring it out like a wet towel. If you're able to twist it so much that the top is now the bottom, it's not a stability or motion-control shoe; it's probably a cushioning shoe. Next, hold the shoe at the heel and forefoot and flex it back. If it only flexes at the toe but doesn't flex at the arch, it probably has more stability or motion-control characteristics. If you flex it back and the shoe bends right at the arch, it's a cushioning shoe. The final test is to feel the midsole, the cushy part of the shoe. If you feel a firm bar on the inside or the outside by the heel, the shoe has stability or motion-control characteristics. If it's the same density the entire way around, and you don't feel any firm plastic bars or posts, it's a cushioning shoe.

As a pedorthist, I have some favorite shoes brands that I recommend to my clients. Because manufacturers often change the model names and numbers, I keep an updated list on my website. You can download it at **thepfplan.com/footwear**.

. . .

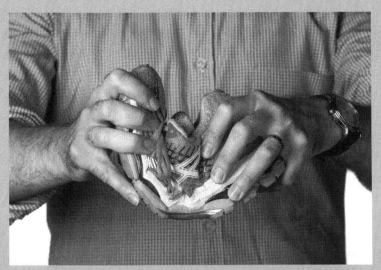

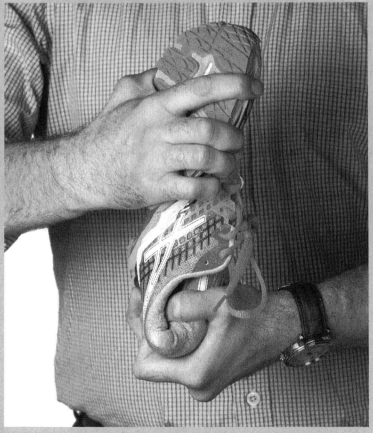

DRESS SHOES

Across all types of footwear, running shoes will give you the most support and cushioning. I strongly urge my plantar fasciitis patients to wear running shoes as much as possible, including to work if at all possible. It's just more comfortable.

Unfortunately, sometimes running shoes just aren't appropriate footwear. In professional and office settings, you may have to wear more formal shoes. Leather soles don't absorb shock very well. Every time your foot hits the ground, the shock is sent into your foot and up the rest of your body to your muscles and your joints. Standing for long periods of time in uncomfortable, leather-soled shoes isn't the most friendly thing for your feet. If you have to wear formal shoes, try to find ones with rubber soles. They'll help dissipate the striking force. They're more forgiving than leather-soled shoes and keep your feet more comfortable over the course of the day. If you have to look professional in an office environment but you want to buy a shoe that's more comfortable, especially if you're walking around a lot all day, look for softer-soled casual dress shoes from companies such as Ecco, Geox, Clarks, Rockport, and Aravon. These are much, much better for your plantar fasciitis than wearing traditional leather-soled dress shoes.

A lot of my female patients tell me their feet hurt less when they wear high heels. The reason for that is because wearing a high heel shifts most of the pressure onto the ball of your foot; you're taking it off the heel. I don't have a problem with my women clients wearing heels if they need to look professional at work. Especially if you mostly sit for your work, what you're wearing on your feet doesn't have as huge a bearing as it would if you spent the day on your feet (minus affecting forefoot conditions, but that's an entire other book). I'm much more concerned with what you're wearing before you go to work, after you come home, on the weekend, and when you're active. Even so, high heels bring their own foot problems. I recommend low-heeled shoes, 13 mm or lower, for women's dress shoes whenever possible.

I tell my patients that when it comes to footwear, if you can do the best-case scenario 90 percent of the time, what you do for the other 10 percent, when life happens and you have to wear silly shoes, is basically inconsequential. It's not going to make a big difference. You might be a bit sorer while doing it, but you won't be doing any lasting harm.

WORK SHOES

I have a patient who calls his work boots Satan's footwear. He's not the only one who complains that work boots make their feet hurt. Work boots are basically meant to protect your feet against crush and puncture injuries if something falls on your foot. The green triangle on the boot means it has a steel toe and a steel shank and meets CSA standards (the US equivalent is boots that are OSHA-certified). Work boots are also rated for other things, such as static and slip, but the primary purpose is still to avoid crush and puncture injuries.

I've found that the real money in making a work boot goes into the safety features. It doesn't go into features that make your feet as comfortable as they could be, because to make a work boot that is both safe and comfortable is expensive. Most are one or the other, unless you want to spend upward of $200. I can pretty much guarantee that cheaper boots won't be geared toward comfort.

To get more comfort from your work boots, I recommend removing the sock liner that comes with it. (Sock liner is just another way of saying insole.) The sock liner that comes in your new boots may be paper-thin, probably no more than 1 or 2 mm thick. Sock liners that are too thin offer no cushioning or support. Try to replace your current boots with a pair that come with a sock liner that's as thick, cushy, and supportive as possible. Look for one that's at least 6 mm thick right from the manufacturer, before you add anything. Be careful when stuffing your current boot full of more cushioning. If the original sock liner was very thin, it might affect the boots' ability to protect against crush injury.

HIKING BOOTS

Hiking boots come up over the ankle and are designed to give you more ankle support than a running shoe. Some people with plantar fasciitis find them a bit more comfortable. If you have a medium to lower type of arch and you want to get lots of stability, then a hiking boot makes a lot of sense, because you lace it up to above the ankle. There's more shoe around your foot, so there's more to give you overall support. Typically, hiking boots have soles that are a bit stiffer than a running shoe. The stiffer sole gets you to work less. You can't bend your toes back as much, which reduces the strain in your plantar fascia, which can help to make things better. If you like hiking boots and you don't mind wearing them day-to-day, they're actually great footwear if you have plantar fasciitis. The drawback to a hiking boot is that you usually don't get as much cushioning as you do in a running shoe. It's a matter of trying both types of shoe on and seeing which one gives you the most comfort right off the bat. Some people want that biomechanical control of their feet to reduce stress and strain on the soft tissues. Other people want cushioning for the area around their heel where it hurts. It comes down to what feels best to you.

CHAPTER 10

TRY OFF-THE-SHELF ORTHOTICS

The T in REST stands for try, as in try off-the-shelf orthotics. The word "orthotic" comes from the Greek root *ortho*, meaning to straighten or align. An orthotic is an externally applied device used to modify the structural or functional characteristics of the human skeleton. Another way to define an orthotic is it's a device that aids in the movement or support of a body part. A back brace is an orthotic. A wrist brace is an orthotic. As a pedorthist, I customize or design orthotics that fit into your shoes to support your feet and ankles. If you have a typical case of plantar fasciitis, however, you don't usually need me to make *custom* orthotics for you if you're in the acute phase (weeks 1 through 4) and before you've really tried the REST protocol. You can buy effective off-the-shelf orthotics at any well-stocked pharmacy, specialty shoe store, or from your local foot specialist. There are always exceptions to the rule, though.

The goal of an orthotic, whether off-the-shelf or custom, is to improve your comfort and reduce compensation and the likelihood of a secondary injury. In my extensive experience, just about everyone with plantar fasciitis can benefit from trying an orthotic. In particular, if you stand or walk on hard surfaces for long periods of time, or if you have really low- or high-arched feet, I suggest trying off-the-shelf orthotics as soon as you're diagnosed with PF.

GETTING THE RIGHT FIT

Any well-stocked pharmacy or specialty shoe store will have a good selection of off-the-shelf foot orthotics that may be helpful. Heel gel pads and cups, for instance, can help relieve pain by cushioning the impact on your heel and raising your heel up slightly to take some of the stress off your foot. You can also try cushioning insoles. With these products, some trial and error may be needed to find something that works well for you.

Just as shoe manufacturers design their shoes using lasts that are that company's idea of a normal human foot, so do manufacturers of orthoses. Your foot isn't always going to match up to the contour of that off-the-shelf device. The arch contour is made to fit the average arch. If you have an arch that's really high or really low, you could actually have more pain if you try to wear an off-the-shelf device where the contours hit your foot in the wrong way or put load on your foot in a way that's uncomfortable. That's why when I recommend off-the-shelf devices, I recommend the kind that are heat moldable. They're the closest thing to having your orthotics custom-made. These aren't usually found in pharmacies, but you can easily buy them online (check my website at **thepfplan.com/shop**) or at specialty shoe stores.

Heat-moldable orthotics are quick and simple to personalize for an excellent fit. You put them in the oven at a low temperature for just a minute or two. Put the orthotic into your shoe, put the shoe on your foot (wear socks), and then stand for a minute or so. The orthotic molds to your foot so that you get a contour that matches up with it. One thing we know for sure about orthotics is that comfort is the greatest predictor of success with them. If they're not comfortable, you just won't wear them.

If you have a really low or really high arch, you might need custom orthotics. But for most people, I recommend starting with the simplest, easiest, least expensive, and most convenient approach. It makes sense to try the low-cost alternative first in the early stages. If you want to know if a custom orthotic device is going to work well, try the off-the-shelf ones first. If they help but not enough, chances are good that custom orthotics will help you as well. If you get some relief but not enough relief, then that might be a good indication you need to go see a foot specialist. If you get no relief or the orthotic makes you worse, it could just be that the device was matched really poorly to your foot. Seeking professional help to find out whether or not an orthotic is going to work for you is a good idea.

For people with more typical feet, the likelihood that heat-moldable orthotics will give you full relief is hard to predict. It's different for everybody. Some people will get enough relief from following the REST protocol and adding in the orthotic that their plantar fasciitis is going to subside. For others, REST plus an off-the-shelf orthotic will only get them to around 60 percent better. That's when they come to see me so that I can make them something customized that gets them the rest of the way to pain free.

Knowing how to measure the foot properly is key to fitting orthotics properly. You want the orthotic to fit to your arch length, not your heel-to-toe length. Let's say you're a size 9 shoe. You might actually be a size 11 off-the-shelf device. You want to step on it and make sure that the arch contour of the device matches your arch contour. Most of the time, your arch length is longer than your heel-to-toe length. You have to buy a bigger orthotic and then cut it to fit your shoe properly. For more information on how to get your orthotics to fit exactly right, see our guide at **thepfplan.com/OTS**.

CHOOSING OFF-THE-SHELF ORTHOTICS

The foot care section of the pharmacy can be confusing because you have a lot of different types of off-the-shelf orthotics from which to choose. Use the following chart to help you figure out what the best choice for you would be.

Type of Orthotic	Description	Pros	Cons
Heel Cups	• Soft-cushioned heel cups or lifts that are placed under the heel	• More cushioning under the heel. • Inexpensive •Fits most shoes	• No arch support • May make heel lift and slip • Do not move pressure from heel into arch
Soft Arch	• A soft-cushioned insole • Most Dr. Scholl's insoles fit this description	• Better cushioning than the sock liner in current shoe. • Inexpensive •Fits most shoe types	• Low to no support • Can be bulky • Not fitted to foot. Lifespan is only 3 months*
Fixed arch	• Plastic shell that is molded to fit the average arch • Superfeet and PowerStep are good representations	• Depending on your arch, some will get good arch support • Inexpensive • Fits most shoe types	• Low cushioning compared to soft arch– depending on your arch, can fit well or cause pain • Lifespan is 6 months*
Heat-molded	• The orthotic is heated and placed into shoes to mold to the foot • Brings the ground closer to the foot • Sole is our favorite brand	• Better arch contour. Lower chance of new pain due to bad fit • Can be a good blend of cushioning and support	• Bulky for some shoes– user error in molding can lead to poor fit • Lifespan is 6–12 months*

* Lifespan is estimated and may be more or less depending on user weight and activity level.

ORTHOTIC PROS AND CONS

The pro of an orthotic is that if it's going to help you, you'll know pretty quickly because you'll have less pain soon after you start wearing it. You'll be able to put more pressure on your arch, which takes some of the pressure off your heel, so you'll feel better when you're walking. You're going to have a faster recovery, and you may not have the expense of going with a custom device.

The con to off-the-shelf orthotics is they can be quite bulky. They can make you worse if they're not properly fit, and they wear out relatively quickly. An off-the-shelf device might only last you for a couple weeks if you're a heavy marathon runner. If your activity is only light to moderate, the orthotic might last six to eight months, especially if you're overweight. Eight months is pretty much the limit, though. By then the orthotic has flattened out and lost its ability to provide support and cushioning. Throw them away and get new ones.

ARE THEY HELPING?

Once you start using an orthotic, track how you feel. They should be helping, not hurting you. (I know this sounds like simple advice, but you'd be surprised how often I hear people say that they continued to wear an orthotic even though it was uncomfortable.)

HOW DO THEY WORK?

I'm an expert on foot orthotics, yet if you were to ask me why do orthotics work or how do feet work, the answer at the end of the day is that we don't really know. We used to think that any movement of the foot that wasn't in a neutral position, meaning a position where it's neither over-pronated or over-supinated, was the cause of all foot pathology. The problem with that theory is it was never empirically validated. It wasn't until the mid-1990s that it was finally disproven. The problem now is that we don't know what to replace it with. At this point, there are eight different competing theories as to how the foot actually works, but no one theory has won out over the others yet (Lee 2001). Researchers are making great strides toward understanding how your feet work, but it's still a huge area of uncertainty. I believe that right now, biomechanical research just isn't sensitive enough to be able to see all of the small articulations deep in the foot and to quantify them accurately using 3-D motion analysis. A new field of motion study based on X-rays (fluoroscopy) may give us the answers we're looking for. To get an idea of what that looks like, visit solescience. ca/research, or read the paper by Balsdon et al., 2016 referenced in the bibliography. (Full disclosure, I was the foot specialist involved in this research.)

WHEN SHOULD YOU START FEELING BETTER?

At a minimum, you'll need to do the REST protocol for six weeks. By the end of those six weeks, you're going to be in one of two different groups: responding well, or not. If you're responding to the REST protocol well, you should feel 70–100 percent better than when you began. If you're not responding well, you won't even be at 20 or 30 percent. If you're at the 70 percent or greater, hang in there and keep doing the stretches. You might just need a bit more time to heal. If every week the pain is getting better than the week before, then continue on. If you're not getting better, or if you've plateaued at an unacceptably high pain level, then perhaps you need to move on to Phase 2 (see chapter 13).

RATE YOUR PAIN

Progress can be slow in healing plantar fasciitis. Sometimes it's hard to realize that you're getting better. I suggest keeping track of how you feel on a weekly basis. You'll be able to see if you're progressing or not. This is useful information for you, and it's also helpful for your health-care provider.

To do this, use the chart at right or take a sheet of paper and put two headings on it: week and morning pain. At the end of the first week of following the REST protocol, write down week 1 and then rate your morning pain from that week on a scale of 0 to 10. Zero means no pain; 10 means the worst pain. Continue to note your pain level at the end of each week for at least the next five weeks and preferably until you reach zero for a few weeks running.

As the weeks go by, you should see that your morning pain is gradually diminishing, which is a sure sign that you're getting better. If you've hit a plateau and aren't really improving week over week, you'll be able to see that as well. If you're not seeing improvement each week, maybe it's time to think about moving on to the next level of treatment.

Week #	Morning Pain										
Week 1	0	1	2	3	4	5	6	7	8	9	10
Week 2	0	1	2	3	4	5	6	7	8	9	10
Week 3	0	1	2	3	4	5	6	7	8	9	10
Week 4	0	1	2	3	4	5	6	7	8	9	10
Week 5	0	1	2	3	4	5	6	7	8	9	10

CHAPTER 11

SECONDARY COMPLICATIONS

W hen you have plantar fasciitis, you're at greater risk of a secondary complication. Fortunately, there are things you can do to avoid injuring other areas because of plantar fasciitis.

The most common secondary complaint I see with plantar fasciitis is pain on the outside part of the foot. Because your plantar fascia starts on the inside part of your heel, when it hurts, you unconsciously shift pressure from that area to try to protect it. You end up shifting your weight onto the outside part of your foot. It doesn't take long for compensation to lead to pain. This is another important reason to begin treatment early.

The problem is that the bones on the outside of your foot are much smaller. They're not meant to be loaded in the same way as the bones on the inside of your foot. It's easy to start hurting both the bone structure on the outside of your foot and the soft tissue structures. The tendons and muscles can become overused because they're compensating for the change in your gait and trying to keep that part of your foot stable. I see over-compensation injuries that include pain on the outside of the foot, pain on the outside of the ankle and knee, and hip and back pain, all because of walking differently due to plantar fasciitis. I even sometimes see stress fractures from a patient changing how he or she runs to compensate for the PF. Everything that we're doing in the REST protocol is trying to prevent secondary complications. If you now have pain in another area, or even more than one area, you may have a secondary injury. If it's a nagging, low-grade pain that lasts for longer than a couple of days, chances are it's related to the primary problem of plantar fasciitis. Talk to your health-care professional.

HOW TO AVOID SECONDARY INJURY

In my opinion, the best way to avoid injuring another area on your body is to follow the REST protocol to reduce your morning pain as much as possible. Make sure your footwear fits well and is as comfortable as possible. Get an orthotic into that footwear that will allow you to put as much normal pressure on your foot as you would with everyday activity. Really pay attention to any change in your gait. Look at your foot now and then as you walk. Often you can actually see that you've started walking on the outside of your foot. If you don't notice it, someone else might. Often a patient tells me that his or her spouse was the first to notice that the patient was walking funny and asked what was wrong.

If you realize that your gait is really different as a result of your plantar fasciitis, it might be time to see a health-care professional. It might be time to move to Phase 2 of treatment. In my practice, the people with secondary injuries have gone through Phase 1 and it hasn't helped. They've been compensating on their foot for anywhere between six and twelve weeks. By that point, we're dealing with secondary injuries on top of the plantar fasciitis. Now they have both ankle tendinitis and plantar fasciitis! It's much more difficult to heal both problems together. Avoiding secondary injury is a much better approach.

If you can see or feel that you're compensating, being active in something that is physically demanding on your lower body is probably not a good idea. Adding compensation on top of activity, where you're demanding more from your body, is just asking for one of your secondary injuries to come up.

ASSISTIVE DEVICES

Assistive devices such as canes can be very helpful for people with plantar fasciitis, especially if they're older. As you age, the fat pad at the bottom of your heel naturally thins. The plantar fascia can also become more brittle with age, and without the cushioning the fat pad provides, the origin of the plantar fascia is at risk of injury. That helps explain why elderly people get plantar fasciitis. At the same time, elderly people have much less ability to compensate in their gait, which puts them at greater risk of falling and developing serious secondary injuries, such as a sore knee or much worse, a broken hip. Assistive devices such as canes, walkers, and rolling walkers help patients walk without compensating. Using a cane or a walker might seem intuitive and simple, but in many ways, it isn't. If you feel you'd like to try an assistive device, get professional guidance from a physical or occupational therapist about which device is best for you and how to use it.

In general, compensation and variability when we walk is a good thing. It allows us to adapt to uneven terrain and avoid falls. We know that too much variability or too little variability can be bad. But if an injury such as plantar fasciitis makes your gait be over-constrained, you lose that variability. That increases your risk of falling. It's an important reason to make every effort to treat your plantar fasciitis.

CHAPTER 12

ICING

S ince PF is a condition that goes through stages from acute (inflammatory) to chronic (degradation), or perhaps a combination of the two, icing your painful foot is one of those treatments that will either help you find some relief, or won't help at all. The only way to know is to try it.

Icing works best if you start doing it right away, when the plantar fasciitis has only just been injured and is in the first few days of the acute phase. At that point, the plantar fascia is probably inflamed. Icing can help bring down the swelling inflammation causes, which helps to relieve the pain. If you've acutely injured your foot or if you've heard a snap or a pop or felt anything that makes you think maybe you've ruptured your plantar fascia, start icing it right away (unless you have a condition like Raynaud's syndrome or poor circulation in your feet, where icing is contraindicated).

If you've had PF for so long that it's become chronic, icing is less likely to help. By now, the pain is coming more from tissue degradation than from inflammation. In my experience, if you've had plantar fasciitis for less than seven months, icing may be helpful. If it's been going on for longer than that, icing probably won't help. Even so, if you came to me after having PF for nine months, I would still suggest giving icing a try. At the end of the working day, or after long periods of activity, or if you're on your feet on hard surfaces throughout the day, icing might still provide some relief. I recommend doing it not just at home but also at work if possible, during your lunch break if you can.

With icing, we're aiming for two different effects. If you have the inflammatory type of planner fasciitis, icing works to reduce the inflammation. It's helping with pain control by reducing inflammation and also just numbing the area a bit. It's also helping with blood flow. As you start icing, the blood vessels contract. When you stop and the area warms up again, that encourages blood flow to come back to the area. The plantar fascia is poorly vascularized, so helping with that is only a good thing.

HOW TO ICE

It's hard to wrap an ice bag around your foot. You don't really want to do that anyway—you want the cold to be applied just to the plantar fascia. A simple, inexpensive way to do this is to fill a plastic water or soda bottle about two-thirds full of water and put it in the freezer. When you're ready to ice, take it out and roll your foot over it, from the heel or back part of your arch to the ball of your foot, for ten to fifteen minutes. Repeat several times a day. With the water bottle, you get the benefit of the ice and you also massage the area, which will help as well.

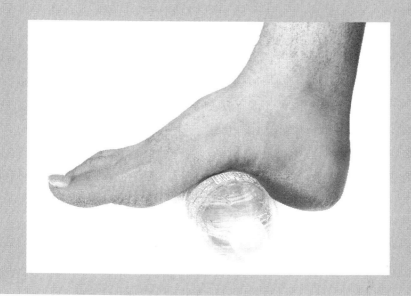

I like the frozen water bottle method, but there are other ways. Some of my patients use frozen golf balls. Some people just put an ice pack or a bag of frozen peas on their heels. Some people tell me they fill a bucket with icy water and stick the lower third of their foot, from the heel to the arch, into it. Experiment and find a way that works comfortably for you. You could also try the Sole-Mender, a frozen ice massager invented by Ehan Kamat when he was only thirteen. He's one of the most articulate, inventive young entrepreneurs of his generation. Ehan developed this machine for his mother to provide pain relief combining ice and tissue massage while she was suffering through PF. Details about this awesome solution to the ice/massage combo are at solemender.com.

If icing works for you, great—keep it up. If it doesn't, you'll know in a few days. Move on.

Some of my patients like to do contrast baths. Start with a bucket of hot (not really hot) water and a bucket of ice water. Put your painful foot into the ice water and keep it there as long as you can tolerate it. Then put your foot into the hot water and move it around for a couple of minutes or longer if you can stand it. Repeat as often as you can bear it, ending in the ice water. The idea here is you're making the blood vessels constrict (vasoconstriction) in the cold water and then expand (vasodilation) in the hot water. End in the cold. You squeeze the blood flow out in the cold and then open up the vessels and promote the blood flow back in the hot. Some people swear this helps; others say it doesn't do anything except make a mess in the bathroom. Try it and see for yourself.

WHO SHOULDN'T ICE

Icing is worth trying and may really help, but some people shouldn't do it. If you have high blood pressure or any sort of circulation problem in your feet or legs, such as peripheral artery disease, don't ice. If you have any sort of reduced sensation in your feet or legs, don't ice. If you have diabetic neuropathy in your feet, don't ice. If you have Raynaud's syndrome, don't ice. And if you just hate the feeling of icing, you don't have to do it.

HEAT INSTEAD

Just as some people benefit from icing and others don't, some people benefit from warmth on their foot. I don't know of any studies about using heat for PF, but some patients tell me it just makes their foot feel better. At the end of the day, if you feel better while you're giving your foot some warmth, I'm not going to say it's wrong. It's worth trying. However, don't use a heating pad or a therapeutic heat pack if you have any sort of circulation problem or reduced sensation in your feet. Don't use heat if you have diabetic neuropathy.

MOVING ON

You've followed the REST protocol for at least six weeks. Chances are good that you're feeling a lot better. Let's look at your pain on a "percentage of better" scale. If you're 80 percent better or more and are seeing consistent improvement week after week (as noted in the pain chart in chapter 7), you probably need to stick with the protocol for a few more weeks, until you've healed completely. Once you're pain free, your next step is to keep your plantar fasciitis from coming back. To learn how to do that, skip to Part V: Prevention. If you're interested in having my team help you implement the stages of this book, please visit **thepfplan.com/yourteam** to find out how we can work with you one-on-one to personalize your treatment plan.

But what if you've felt some improvement, but now things have stalled out at an unacceptably high pain level? If you haven't seen consistent improvement, are below 80 percent better at this point, or have started to notice new pain elsewhere from compensation, it's time to move on to Phase 2. Keep reading.

MEDICATION

Nonprescription medications have their place in treating plantar fasciitis. I'm not a medical doctor, however, so I don't feel qualified to discuss medication. Fortunately, my colleague Dr. Tatiana Jevremovic, MD, CCFP(EM), dip sport med sport and exercise medicine physician at the Fowler Kennedy Clinic is a medical doctor. She's agreed to shed some light on the topic.

Anti-Inflammatory Drugs

According to Dr. Jevremovic, over-the-counter nonsteroidal anti-inflammatory drugs (NSAIDs) such as aspirin, ibuprofen (Advil, Motrin), and naproxen (Aleve) can help reduce pain by reducing inflammation and swelling. They don't help everyone, but they're worth trying to see if you're a responder. Use these medications with caution. Even at low doses, they can cause side effects such as gastrointestinal bleeding, stomach pain, hypertension, kidney disease, and allergic reactions. Talk to your doctor before you try these for plantar fasciitis.

If you can't take NSAIDs because they upset your digestion or you're allergic, you can try acetaminophen (Tylenol). Unless you're allergic to it, this drug is usually very safe. It doesn't have the anti-inflammatory properties that NSAIDs do, however, so it may not help much.

Topical creams that contain NSAIDs are an alternative. The advantage is that the drug is absorbed into the skin above the painful area, instead of having to go through your digestive system. As with pills, however, there's no clear evidence that any of the creams work.

**Consult your doctor or pharmacist
before seeking medications.**

PART THREE

TREATMENT PHASE 2: ORTHOSES

CUSTOM-MADE ORTHOTICS

You've done everything suggested in the REST protocol for six weeks or more, and you're still not making progress. You're either not seeing week-on-week progression, or you're actually worse. Don't despair. Your next step (OK, can't help making that pun) is to visit someone like me for custom-made orthotics.

The world of custom-made orthotics is confusing for consumers—it's like the Wild West! Lots of different types of practitioners (some are not even foot specialists) claim to make "the best" custom orthotics, based on many different theories and using a lot of different materials. Custom orthotics can be expensive, so I want to help you understand how to make the best choices and to get custom orthotics that really help.

First, custom-made orthotics can truly be helpful, but they need to made correctly so that they fit your feet exactly. When you choose a provider, look for someone who has been formally trained in building custom-made foot orthotics, such as a pedorthist. Be skeptical of someone whose training was a weekend course, or who does custom-made orthotics as a side business or offers you a free assessment. Be wary of someone who has the front desk staff doing assessments and taking foot molds.

For an orthotic to be truly custom, we start with a 3-D cast or impression of your foot. That's usually done using foam, plaster, wax, or a laser light scan. A 2-D pressure pattern done just by taking a footprint (digital or ink) of your foot is not enough. Due to variations in human feet, using 2-D images to make a 3-D product is not the most effective approach. We don't have an X + Y = Z formula for making orthotics. There's a huge amount of individual variability among feet. What works for one person isn't going to work for somebody else. Your orthotics need to be made and adjusted for your individual comfort. Be patient with your practitioner and with the outcome. It may take a little time to get the orthotics just right for your feet.

In my opinion, an effective orthotic for plantar fasciitis places as much pressure into your arch as you can tolerate, while also removing pressure from your heel with softer cushioning. Your orthotics should fit well right from the start, but it's still important to break them in slowly so your body has a chance to adjust to the change. I recommend wearing them for just half the day for the first few days and then wearing them a little longer each day until you're comfortable with them all day long. Ultimately, you want to be wearing your orthotics as much as possible.

Research suggests that comfort is the greatest predictor of success with orthotics (Mils et al. 2012; Mills et al. 2012; Mündermann et al. 2002). If your orthotic isn't comfortable, *take it back to be adjusted.* Remember the princess and the pea? You might just be the princess.

Orthotics only work as well as the shoes you put them into—check back to chapter 9 on finding the best shoes for you. Once placed in your shoes, orthotics shouldn't hurt. They'll feel new and different at first, but they should never be uncomfortable or painful. (If they didn't feel different, you'd have to wonder what we're doing for you.) To get the most out of them, wear the new orthotics in your shoes first thing in the morning, after you've done the stretching part of the REST protocol. Make sure that your first few steps of the day are done with your shoes on and orthotic in.

CHAPTER 13

CUSTOM-MADE ORTHOTICS

C ustom-made orthotics are devices placed in your shoe to help relieve pressure and provide cushioning and support for your foot. They can be very, very helpful for relieving the symptoms of plantar fasciitis, but they're not always necessary. If you've done the REST protocol and you're feeling 80 percent or more better, give yourself some more time, preferably another two to three weeks, to see if you get any more improvement. If you're really close to being 100 percent, don't jump into custom orthotics right away. Continue with the REST protocol. But if you've stalled in your progress or feel you're going backward, then it's important to see a specialist who can talk to you about custom orthotics.

It's difficult to estimate how many people will have to move from REST into custom orthotics. Based on my clinical experience, I find that somewhere between 30 and 40 percent of people need to progress beyond REST. People over age forty make up the majority of that group. Younger athletes will typically recover faster.

Another reason for seeking custom orthotics before completing the REST protocol is that you're starting to feel sore in other areas because you're compensating for the pain by changing how you move. Your heel has been sore for a couple of months and now the outside of your foot or the ball of your foot hurts, or your knee or your hip is getting sore. Now it's time to think about custom orthotics while continuing the REST protocol. If you have an additional condition, such as diabetes or osteoarthritis, you might want to talk to a specialist about custom orthotics right away to help prevent secondary injury.

Sometimes I'll have a patient who has had symptoms for more than seven months but hasn't done anything about them. In those cases, I recommend REST and a custom orthotic simultaneously. That's because we know that people who go untreated for over seven months have a smaller likelihood of actually getting better. They need more aggressive treatment.

WHY CUSTOM ORTHOTICS?

Off-the-shelf orthotics, as explained in chapter 10, often help with plantar fasciitis. They're a generic solution that often works for the average person. If you're not average, though, an off-the-shelf orthotic just won't fit your foot properly, or you might need greater correction than an off-the-shelf product can provide. That's where custom-made orthotics come in. These devices are made specifically for your foot using a 3-D cast.

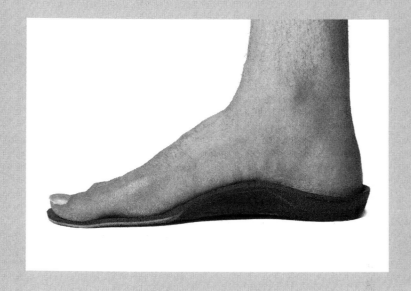

A custom-made orthotic can give you all the individual support, stability, and cushioning you need. In some ways, the sky's the limit. We have all kinds of options for materials, shapes, and styles. Because they're fully custom, they can be made to fit any kind of foot. Custom-made orthotics are also fully adjustable if things don't feel quite right.

Confusingly, another type of orthotic is called customized or custom-prescribed devices. These usually are not made from a 3-D cast of the foot. They're usually done with 2-D methods.

The difference is huge. In terms of price, there's often little to distinguish the two. Customized orthotics really aren't that different from a well-made, off-the-shelf device. Custom-made orthotics fit the contours of the feet exactly. They're designed to offer you the best kind of support, control, and cushioning. Orthotics can be expensive. If you're spending anywhere between $400 and $600 on a device, you want to know that it is truly custom-made for you, not something that's just kind of close to custom-made.

TYPES OF CUSTOM-MADE ORTHOTICS

A fully custom-made orthotic can be one of two different types: Accommodative or corrective. An accommodative device essentially builds the ground up to your foot. It's designed to be the best match of your foot and to redistribute pressures on the bottom part of your foot. This type of orthotic is best for people who need the pressure redistributed, but without lots of corrective support. Accommodative custom-made orthotics aren't trying to move your foot into a better position or encourage a different range of motion. People who have diabetic complications, have certain types of arthritis, or have fixed bony deformities would need this sort of device.

Corrective custom-made orthotics try to guide or "correct" your foot into a different position or mechanical pattern. For example, let's say you have really low arches that collapse when you walk and thus place more strain on your plantar fascia. Corrective orthotics try to decrease the amount that your arch falls and thus decrease the strain on your plantar fascia.

Corrective orthotics have been extensively studied for plantar fasciitis. Typically, they're made of a hard material that tries to push your foot into the "correct position." But what if I told you that the correct position for your foot *doesn't actually exist?* This is the problem that all of us who make custom foot orthotics face. I don't like to make everyone fit into one box or one idea about what's "correct." One person might feel a lot better with a ton of support, while someone else needs very little support but more cushioning. Individuality plays such a huge role that I can't say that any one style of orthotic is the best (and the research doesn't, either!).

I can say that in general, someone with a lower arch type of foot that's very mobile is putting excessive strain on their soft tissues. A corrective device to reduce the strain on the soft tissues from that extra mobility would probably help. Someone with a higher arch foot will have a stiff, immobile, inflexible foot. That means people with a higher arch are putting lots of pressure and load on their plantar fascia just at the origin point. Their arch is so high they put a lot of pressure on their heels and their forefeet. For these people, trying to off-load the pressure is usually the better approach.

No matter what the type, to get the orthotic exactly right takes a little trial and error. It's really more an iterative process. We have a pretty good idea of where to start; it's just getting the fit exactly right that can take some time and revision. We see how the patient responds to the orthotic as an individual and then adjust course. I can treat two people with the exact same foot type and the exact same problem, and they wind up with drastically different orthotics.

Why is that? We all have receptors in the skin of our feet that are sensitive to pressure, touch, vibration, heat, and cold. Some people have more of these receptors per square inch and some people have fewer. If you have more, you're probably more sensitive to what's happening on the bottom part of your foot. If you have more receptors per square inch, and I put something in your shoe that presses into the bottom of your foot, you might perceive that to be much more uncomfortable than somebody who has fewer receptors. The problem is that we can't really predict who's going to be able to get used to that feeling and who's not. We just have to try and see what happens.

WHO SHOULD MAKE YOUR ORTHOTIC?

You definitely want a certified professional or a trained practitioner to build your custom-made orthotics. This usually means somebody with some type of post-graduate training specifically in both of the design and the manufacture of custom foot orthotics. A Canadian-certified pedorthist has one full year of training, or more than 1,200 hours, in custom-made foot orthotics and footwear design and manufacture—on top of four years of undergraduate training. Podiatrists and chiropodists are trained in the design, but not necessarily the manufacture, of orthotics. In the United States, pedorthists must have a minimum of 1,000 hours of training beyond their pedorthic precertification education course. In my view, you should always work with someone who is trained specifically in this area. A practitioner who has taken a weekend course doesn't have adequate training to fit you well.

When you're choosing a practitioner to make your custom orthotics, look for people with the right initials after their names. That would be C.Ped or C.Ped (C) if they're a certified pedorthist in Canada. It would be DPM for podiatrist and DCH for a chiropodist. In Canada, CO means a certified orthotist. In the United States, the professionals who can provide orthotics vary by state.

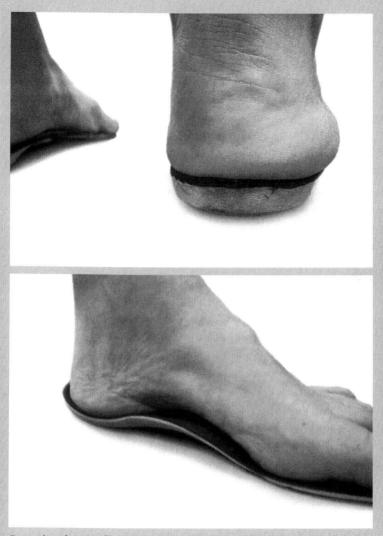

Examples of poorly-fitting orthotics made by an untrained provider—
BUYER BEWARE! Notice how the foot does not fit.

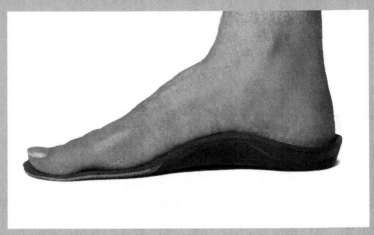

*An example of a proper fitting orthotic. Notice the fit in the arch—
it matches perfectly.*

I'm a pedorthist. That's probably a new word for you! We're a
small, but growing group of professionals who are foot orthotic
and orthopedic footwear experts. A pedorthist is one of the few
health-care professionals trained in the assessment of lower-limb
anatomy and muscle and joint function. With specialized education
and training in foot orthotics and footwear, Canadian-certified
pedorthists help to alleviate pain, abnormalities, and debilitating
conditions of the lower limbs and feet. Pedorthists are also trained
in *both* the design *and* the manufacture of orthotics. We can see
patients clinically, assess them, and make the right device for them.
Chiropodists and podiatrists can diagnose and assess, but they're
not necessarily trained in how to make orthotics. They'll usually
send a cast of your foot to an outside lab to have them made. Don't
mistake using an external lab as a bad thing, though. The right
external lab can make excellent orthotics. The drawback is that
sometimes it takes a little longer to receive your devices.

WHAT TO ASK

When you visit a foot specialist for orthotics, ask a lot of questions, including the following:

- **Do you make the orthotic?** Some use an external lab to fabricate your orthotics. This can mean a longer lead time just to get them. It can also mean long delays if you need adjustments. The device is sent back to the lab, the adjustment is made, and then it's shipped back to you. The entire process, round-trip, can take as long as four to six weeks. When you're in a lot of pain, that's a long time to wait. A pedorthist usually will make the orthotics on-site and can adjust them quickly in the office. An on-site lab is a plus!

- **Should they hurt?** Definitely not. The best predictor of success with orthotics is comfort. They will feel new and different to your foot, but that doesn't mean you should feel pain. If it hurts, you need an adjustment.

- **Should you have cushioning in the heel?** Yes. The best research and clinical experience tells us the surface area under the heel should be made of a softer material.

- **How long will they last?** Two to four years. The average is somewhere in the middle. If you're heavier or if you run marathons (or both), they'll last closer to the two-year mark. If you're average height and weight and you're exercising only a few times a week, they'll last longer. I've had patients go as long as nine years with the same orthotics before they needed to be replaced, while some needed new ones as quickly as eleven months.

- **Will you take a 3-D cast or mold of my foot?** The answer here should always be yes. A 3-D shape always needs to be taken for custom-made orthotics. A 2-D footprint is not sufficient to make a truly custom device.

HOW DO CUSTOM ORTHOTICS WORK?

How orthotics work is a really fun topic for me, because I'm an adjunct research professor in the school of physical therapy at Western University in London. When I ask this question of my students, I get a variety of answers. Most commonly, students suggest that they work by controlling biomechanics, or by optimizing the foot position, or by decreasing pressures to optimal levels. Every year, my students are horrified when I say, "These are all great answers, but at the end of the day, we really don't know, definitively, how these things work." I tell them the better question is, "Are orthotics effective to treat different kinds of foot pathologies?"

A lot of research shows that orthotics are in fact effective to treat foot pain, it just can't say why. Ever since a podiatrist named Merton L. Root, DPM published a textbook on the late 1950s that said the foot functions best when it's in a neutral position— neither supinated or pronated—we were taught that if the foot deviated from this position, that was the biomechanical reason for foot injuries. The thinking was that if the foot was abnormal, there had to be a "normal" standard.

The problem with that theory is that I see people every day with "abnormal" but pain-free feet. If you look at these pictures of two of my patients, you'll see that in the inset photo, the arch is very, very low. In fact, the full arch touches the ground—this person has flat feet. In the main picture, the arch is "normal." According

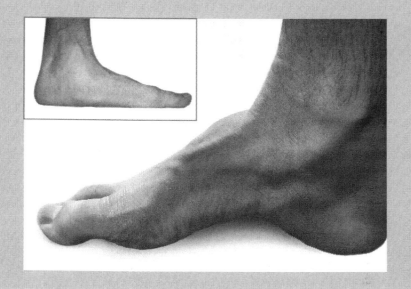

to Dr. Root, the person with flat feet should be very susceptible to injury. The problem is that of these two people, the person with the really low arch is a marathon runner who's never had a foot problem in his life. The person with the normal arch has all kinds of pain and problems. Although the neutral position theory was never actually scientifically validated, it continued to be taught until the mid-1990s, when a group of researchers studied it. They wanted to get a better idea of what was really happening. What they found was that the neutral position doesn't actually hold true for everybody who doesn't have pain. That led to eight competing theories to explain foot injuries, none of which has been proven to be the "right" one.

Of those eight competing theories, the one that I think makes the most sense is called soft tissue stress theory (we covered why in chapter 4). This approach elegantly answers the question, How can some people have very pronated feet and never have problems, while others have "normal" feet and have all sorts of problems?

Soft tissue stress theory says that the soft tissues of different people have natural variation within the normal range. Some people have soft tissues that are better able to withstand more cyclical soft tissue loading than others. That might explain why someone with a super-low arch may not have any pain, whereas someone with a normal-looking foot does. The normal foot has a smaller range within the soft tissues; it's more subject to increased trauma under stress.

If we say that some people have a greater ability to deal with soft tissue stress and some people have less, we can put people on an injury spectrum. We see some on the far left of the spectrum who are able to do everything "wrong." They can go from sitting on the couch to running marathons in bad shoes without enough sleep, with poor nutritional habits, and with too-fast training and never get injured. I'm sure you all know that one person, and deep down, we're super jealous of them! At the opposite end of the spectrum is the person who does everything "correctly," wears great shoes, had good training habits, gets great sleep and proper nutrition, but is always hurt.

Most people are somewhere in the middle. The question is where are you? I like to use an Eisenhower matrix to figure this out. If you look at the diagram at right, you'll see that it has four boxes. Soft tissue stress is on the bottom and biomechanics is on the right. If you have really high tolerance to tissue stress and you have really good biomechanics, you might be in that box that doesn't

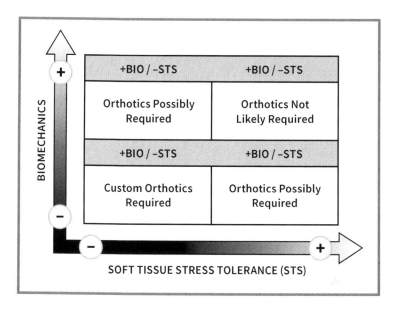

require anything to be done. If you have great biomechanics and you have a poor ability to adapt to tissue stress, you might need to do something, but we're not sure what or how much. The inverse of that is if you have really poor ability to deal with tissue stress and poor biomechanics, then we'll always have to do something for you. If you're in that other box where you've got poor mechanics but a great ability to deal with tissue stress, we might need to do something for you. (I love talking about this stuff, but we do need to discuss other topics. If you want more information, check my website at **thepfplan.com**.)

When we're measuring the foot from a 3-D model perspective in a gait lab, the foot is seen as just going up and down and side to side. In reality, it's much more complicated. The foot has so many moving parts and so many articulations between bones, ligaments, tendons, muscles, and fascii that it can move in a lot of ways. The movements can be so small and subtle that we don't have instruments sensitive enough to detect and measure them without X-ray. Also, footwear plays a big part in obfuscating foot movement and measurement. When someone is wearing shoes, we just can't see what's happening as the foot moves. We're using some new techniques, such as biplanar fluoroscopy, that basically shows you a moving skeleton of the foot that we can then track using other methods.

HOW ARE CUSTOM ORTHOTICS MADE?

How your orthotics are made matters quite a bit. If you haven't responded to the REST protocol, orthotics offer a specifically tailored solution that is modifiable based on your comfort. Orthotics reduce the need to compensate when you walk, which helps you avoid secondary injury.

The best research is divided over the value of custom-made orthotics for plantar fasciitis. One problem with the research is that they all use different styles of orthotics. Add in the variability of feet, and it's very difficult to compare studies. The best clinical evidence tells us that just as feet are variable, so is the response to orthotics. What works for one will not work for another. Working patiently with a qualified provider to find the solution that's best for you is the best approach. My patients tell me every day that their foot orthotics let them live, work, and move with less pain. When they stop wearing the orthotics, their pain returns and their function decreases. Remember, doing nothing and just waiting it out can have potentially more harmful effects than trying something as long as it's not going to hurt.

Just as we have a lot of variability in feet, we also have a lot of variability in an individual's ability to accommodate to the orthotic. That's what makes my work so interesting—and sometimes so frustrating. I never know how someone's going to react to the orthotic until it's under his or her foot. Sometimes we need to go through several rounds of adjustments until it's comfortable. I tell my patients that if the device doesn't need an adjustment, I probably got lucky more than I was skillful.

THE RESEARCH ON ORTHOTICS

Full disclosure: I'm a pedorthist. I'm an orthotics provider. I own an orthotics manufacturing lab. Of course, I'm slightly biased toward using orthotics. That's not to say that I don't listen to the evidence when it's presented to me, but when I do come across a study that says custom-made orthotics aren't an effective treatment for plantar fasciitis, I will critically examine why. For example, one study in 2006 in the prestigious journal Archives of Internal Medicine looked at 135 patients over twelve months and found no difference between the use of over-the-counter or custom-made orthotics (Landorf et al. 2006). Other than methodological problems, such as blinding and confounders, the problem I see with the conclusion is that all the devices used in the study were very hard. If a device is too hard and over-corrective, it may not be comfortable. In that case, it will be ineffective because the patient won't wear it or winds up in more pain due to wearing it. The orthotic ends up in the closet or as a fancy doorstop.

The inverse of the *Archives* study is one from 2006 in *Foot & Ankle International*. This study looked at forty-three patients and followed them over the short and long term (Roos et al. 2006). It found that a soft custom-made orthotic was effective at both improving function and increasing foot-related quality of life, suggesting that foot orthotics are a good choice for the initial treatment of plantar fasciitis (Roos et al. 2006).

In the studies that find orthotics effective, some can point to use of a softer device; the results tend to show decreased pain and increased function. I think it comes down to comfort. The patients in the study were simply able to wear the orthotic regularly and for longer each day.

Due to the *huge* variability in making orthotics, researchers may only conclude that the style of orthotic used in that particular study (and not *all* orthotics in general) may or may not be effective in the treatment of PF. Sadly, some researchers will generalize their findings to "all orthotics" and not just the style they've used.

If you'd like to learn more about the scientific research on foot orthotics, I've got lots of information and discussion on my website at **thepfplan.com/research**.

Since we really don't know how orthotics work, many people still cling to the dogma that hard is better because it holds the foot in the "correct" position. In fact, a great deal of foot orthotics are made using hard substances such as polypropylene plastic. When I see patients who need re-managing of their plantar fasciitis, they almost always tell me that they got orthotics earlier but they wound up in the closet because they hurt too much and they weren't able to be adjusted. That's what I want to avoid at all costs for my patients.

Reed Ferber, a leading researcher in biomechanics at the University of Alberta, published a study in 2015 in *Prosthetics and Orthotics International* that looked at off-the-shelf and heat-molded orthotics (Ferber et al. 2015). Ferber found that when these devices were built up to contour the arch, the strain on the plantar fascia was reduced by up to 35 percent. This fits well with the soft tissue stress theory. If you can remove the mechanical stress from the structure, giving it time to heal, that might be why people get better. The orthotic itself doesn't fix plantar fasciitis, it simply gives your foot time to fix itself. I feel Dr. Ferber is very much on the right track here.

In my practice, I build custom orthotics for plantar fasciitis that have some of the firmness of a corrective device in the arch, in combination with a medium-soft cushioning at the heel. I use a plastic material that fills the shape of the arch so that the patient can place as much pressure there as he or she can tolerate, reducing strain of the fascia and producing less strain on the attachment point at the heel. I go one step further by removing all hard plastic under the heel and cushioning with a medium-soft material that can reduce heel pressure by up to 22 percent. This produces a device that is as comfortable as possible. The goal, in my mind, is to reduce the biomechanics that are causing excessive strain with the firm plastic, and to reduce the likelihood of compensation due to pain with the soft cushioning.

Once you get your orthotics, you should see a linear improvement in pain week on week. Continue to track your pain each week as I explained back in chapter 7. If you're not seeing any progress after six weeks, it's possible your orthotics need changing or adjustment. Bring them in. Of course, if the pain gets worse, bring your orthotics in immediately for assessment and adjustment.

Week #	Morning Pain										
Week 1	0	1	2	3	4	5	6	7	8	9	10
Week 2	0	1	2	3	4	5	6	7	8	9	10
Week 3	0	1	2	3	4	5	6	7	8	9	10
Week 4	0	1	2	3	4	5	6	7	8	9	10
Week 5	0	1	2	3	4	5	6	7	8	9	10
Week 6	0	1	2	3	4	5	6	7	8	9	10

* * *

HOW TO WEAR YOUR ORTHOTICS

When we make orthotics, we tell the patient, if you don't break them in slowly, they'll break you in quickly. We don't want that to happen. Depending on the style of orthotics, hard or soft, really corrective, partially corrective, or completely accommodative, the break-in time will vary. Some people can get new orthotics, and they can go all day every day from day one. Some people have to start with half days and try to go a little bit longer each day. Ideally, you'll work up to wearing them 90 percent of your weight-bearing time.

If after half a day your arch is starting to get achy and tired, take them off. You're putting more pressure into an area that isn't used to it anymore. Try again the next day and try to last a little longer. Breaking in orthotics usually takes about seven days. If you've been wearing them for a week and don't love them, bring them back to your specialist.

Because custom-made orthotics alter the movement patterns of your foot and lower limb, the muscles and joints will now move differently. That's going to feel a little bit strange for the first couple of days. Your muscles are going to feel like they've been to the gym. They might feel achy or a bit crampy or sore for the first couple of days. Your calves might feel it the most. That's all normal. The red flag with orthotics is an increase in pain, new pain, or different pain in the first seven days. If any of those things happen, something isn't right. Get back to your specialist.

You might need an adjustment if you get skin irritations or blisters. If you participate in any kind of athletic activity, such as running or basketball, make sure that your devices are comfortable for walking around every day before you wear them for any kind of activity. The last thing you want to do is get orthotics in the morning and go for a 10K run that night. That's the best way to wind up with blisters.

During an adjustment, tell the clinician what the problem is, and then he or she will figure out a way to alter the device. It could be that there's a little bit too much pressure in your arch. There's a really fine line between giving you enough support so that it helps you and giving you too much so that it hurts you. If we need to adjust the amount of arch support, that's very simple. We do it on the spot. I've had people come back for as many as eight adjustments (remember the princess and the pea), but most people will only need one or two. The people who need adjustments really need them. The craziest thing about what I do is that I've seen two millimeters be the difference between someone being able to walk out of my office comfortably or not be able to walk at all because he or she is in pain.

Patients ask me if they can fit an orthotic for plantar fasciitis into a dress shoe. The short answer is only in casual dress shoes meant to take orthotics. The kind of orthotic I advocate for don't works well in leather-soled dress shoes for men or with traditional pumps or higher heels for women. For the orthotic to fit into the shoe, we have to make it so small that it doesn't do any good for plantar fasciitis.

CAN YOU EVER STOP WEARING ORTHOTICS?

Some people worry that they'll develop a dependence on their orthotics. Well, maybe. I view orthotics in two different ways. The

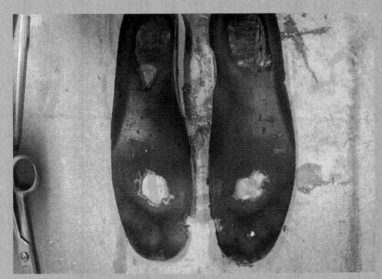
Time for replacements: this was after four years of hard work.

first way is that it's your biomechanics or your foot structure that is the cause of your pain. If that's the case, think of your orthotics as eyeglasses. You'll feel better while you're wearing them; you'll miss them while you're not.

For others, your biomechanics keep you from healing, and the orthotic is a temporary tool to help you feel better. Once you get your foot really strong and healed, then you can wean off of them over time. We can't tell in advance who will be able to graduate from orthotics and who won't.

REPLACING ORTHOTICS

A well-made custom device should last, in the average case, two to three years. Your orthotic might be wearing out and need replacement if you notice that your pain is starting to return. If at the same time you just don't feel the device like you used to, that's the sign that it's time for a replacement. On the other hand, it could be that the orthotic is fine but the shoe is wearing out. Keep an eye on your shoes. A pair of casual dress shoes might last for a couple of years, but if you're a heavy runner, your running shoes might wear out in just a few months. To see if the shoe is wearing out, look at the wear patterns on the sole.

You might also need a replacement if your foot has changed shape recently. After a break, sprain, injury, surgery, or pregnancy, your foot shape can change. If you were doing really well with your orthotic and it suddenly becomes uncomfortable, that usually signals some kind of change. Over time, our foot naturally changes shape and the arch lowers. You'll know that's happened because the orthotic is all of a sudden digging into your arch. Talk to your provider to see if you need a replacement.

CHAPTER 14

NIGHT SPLINTS

For people who aren't responding to orthotic therapy, going to night splints may be necessary. What's a night splint? It's a device that acts as a brace to hold your foot back in a position that gently stretches out your calves and the plantar fascia while you sleep. Some models look a bit like a ski boot cut in half. Some are anterior: they attach in the front of the leg. Others are posterior: they attach at the back of the leg. You can buy these at well-stocked pharmacies and specialty shoe stores, or you can get them online (I carry them through my website).

Night splints stretch your foot and calf, keeping them in an elongated position while you sleep. That keeps your foot from shortening in the night and having the soft tissue start to heal in a relaxed position. By keeping your foot lengthened, when you get up in the morning and take your first few steps, you don't elongate the tissue and end up tearing the half-healing from the night before. That's what all the morning stretches and exercises in the REST protocol are also supposed to do. If you've been doing them and you're still experiencing significant morning pain, then a night splint may be a good option to get a better result first thing in the morning.

You can go to a night splint on your own. Off-the-shelf devices work fine and generally cost under $100. I find that the DonJoy and Ottobock braces work well for most of my patients. You can find these braces at **thepfplan.com/shop**. There's very rarely a reason to have night splints custom-made. Before you try a splint, however, discuss it with the health-care professional who's been managing your case. There might be another approach, such as modifying your orthotics, that should be tried first.

IS A NIGHT SPLINT RIGHT FOR YOU?

You know you should try a night splint if you've been following the REST protocol and wearing custom orthotics for at least twelve weeks and still have pain, especially in the morning. You've added orthotics to the protocol, and while they probably helped somewhat, the pain is still stubbornly there. If you've been faithful about your foot stretches and orthotics and things aren't improving much, don't blame yourself. You're just one of those people who is slow to respond to treatment. Your chances of becoming pain free are still good; it's just going to take longer.

Some experts recommend going to a night splint at the same time you start using orthotics. The evidence suggests that the combination speeds recovery. If you're at 70 percent and making reasonable progress with REST and custom orthotics, you can try using a night splint to speed the healing process up a little bit. This approach won't hurt you, but I don't usually recommend it right away. I feel night splints can be disruptive to your sleep and you shouldn't use them unless you really need them. It's like wearing a boot to bed. The splint itself isn't painful, but it takes a while to get used to wearing it. You can't really sleep comfortably in any position except on your back. Your feet are supposed to be healing while you sleep, but paradoxically, the night splint can keep you from getting the sleep you need. I'd rather try the orthotics alone and maybe make some adjustments to them before moving on to the night splint.

I prefer to use night splints as a fallback for patients who don't respond well to orthotic therapy. The time to decide that is after you've been wearing the orthotic for six to eight weeks. If you're doing really well with the orthotic device—you're 80 percent or more better—it's probably time to modify the orthotic slightly, maybe to give you a little bit more support or perhaps a bit more cushioning, or maybe just a bit more time to be able to get better. As long as you're seeing linear progression and improvement, I think you're OK and don't need to worry about splints. If you're stalled or you're just not progressing, then you can move to a splint.

For chronic plantar fasciitis that has become resistant to treatment, the research tells us that night splints can be very effective. A study published in 1998 in the journal *Foot & Ankle International* suggests that 88 percent of people who tried a night splint responded to treatment, irrespective of foot type, weight, or presence of a heel spur. That's compelling evidence that people who haven't done well with treatment so far might really benefit from a night splint.

ANTERIOR OR POSTERIOR?

A 2012 study in *Foot and Ankle Surgery* suggests that anterior night splints, which attach at the front of the leg, were more effective at reducing pain (Attard and Singh 2012). In seven out of nine cases, the anterior splint reduced pain by 50 percent or more (Attard and Singh 2012). Most of the study participants who wore posterior splints found them uncomfortable, while only 22 percent of those who wore the anterior splints said they were uncomfortable (Attard and Singh 2012). This is interesting, but we have to be cautious about drawing conclusions from a study that only had fifteen participants. If you can't decide between an anterior or posterior splint, maybe you should go with the anterior, based on the study. The study also pointed out the big problem with night splints: they're poorly tolerated. At some point in the night, the splint will get so uncomfortable that you'll take it off.

The researchers suggested that a posterior night splint will keep your foot at about 80–90 degrees. You can extend your foot back even more with this type of splint and pull your toes further toward your shins. Pulling your foot too far back from 90 degrees can be uncomfortable on your Achilles tendon. The researchers concluded that prolonged stretch on your calf and your Achilles is why you end up finding it uncomfortable in the middle of the night and taking it off. Anterior night splints keep your ankle at 90 degrees. It still keeps your foot and your plantar fascia in an extended position to allow the collagen fibers to heal and align themselves in a better position. You're more likely to wear the splint all night long. On a personal note, I've worn both kinds. I definitely find the anterior kind more comfortable.

DEALING WITH NIGHT SPLINTS

By the time you decide to go to a night splint, you're probably twelve to sixteen weeks into the healing journey. If you're not doing better at this point, then we classify you as someone who's just resistant to healing. We don't want your plantar fasciitis to become chronic, so we move you on to trying a night splint.

Like any other treatment, I'd want you to keep it up for six to eight weeks. Continue to do your morning stretches and continue to wear your orthotics. Also, continue to track your pain each week, as explained in chapter 7. As long as you're seeing linear progress, that's positive. If you've plateaued and you're seeing progress again, that's great. Some people will find that the night splint really helps—they may even get to pain free in just a few weeks. Unfortunately, some people find that a night splint just doesn't do anything for them. It's uncomfortable and not helping, and they just don't want to wear it anymore.

Another reason people stop wearing a night splint is that it makes their foot numb. One possible cause is that by dorsiflexing your foot back, you pulled it back too far. Your soft tissue just isn't used to being in that position and gets numb. Posterior splints typically have a triangular foam wedge at the front of the brace that helps to extend your toes back. If you crank your toes back too aggressively, you can place pressure on the small nerves in between the toes, which can cause them to go numb in the middle of the night. If that's the case, try pulling the wedge off.

When you put the splint on at night, you can wear a sock under it if that makes it more comfortable. Be careful not to strap it on too tight. You don't want to pinch your toes or cut off the circulation to your toes or foot. This is especially important if you have diabetes or any sort of impaired circulation to your feet. To check, put on the splint and then pinch the end of your big toe. When you let go, you should see the white area where you pinched turn pink again as the blood supply returns. If it fills slowly, the splint is too tight.

To get a good night's sleep while wearing a night splint, try to make yourself as comfortable as possible with it. Untucking your bed sheets at the foot of the bed is going to make it way easier to get your leg in there while wearing the splint. One really important tip is to remove those expensive, high thread count sheets. The Velcro that holds the splint in place is going to wreck them. Go with some old or inexpensive sheets that you won't mind putting fabric pulls into. If you're really only comfortable when you're sleeping on your stomach, you can try hanging the splinted foot off the end of the bed. You may have some bad nights when you first start wearing the splint, but most people get better at sleeping with it in about a week. Stick it out if you can. Night splints can really help, but some people take much longer than others to see the benefits.

PART FOUR

TREATMENT PHASE 3: EVERYTHING ELSE

INTRODUCTION TO PART FOUR

For some people, Phase 2 treatment still isn't enough to relieve their plantar fasciitis. It's now time to continue with the REST protocol, orthotics, and the other aspects of Phase 2 and move on to Phase 3: trying additional treatments to find something that works.

If you're not making progress with healing your plantar fasciitis despite following the REST protocol, wearing your custom orthotics and night splints, you still have options that can help.

DEALING WITH PAIN AND DEPRESSION

If you're reading this part of the book, there's a good chance you've been living in chronic pain for months. Chronic pain sucks. There's just no better way to say it. I completely understand how distressing it is to have your foot hurt all the time and to not be able to do the things you want to do—I've been there. You may be feeling socially isolated and generally low. I want you to take mental stock of how you really feel.

While there's no universally accepted standard definition of chronic pain, the International Association for the Study of Pain defines it as "pain without apparent biological value that has persisted beyond the normal tissue healing time, usually between three to six months." (IASP 1986) An article in the *British Journal of Psychiatry* suggests that pain is strongly associated with anxiety as well as with depressive disorders (Korff 1996). The pain characteristics that best predict depression are how widespread it is and how much pain interferes with your daily activities (Korff 1996). We know that plantar fasciitis is going to keep you from doing a lot of things. You may not be able to do something as simple as walking the dog or going for a walk with a friend or spouse, let alone being able to spend eight to ten hours of your day at work standing on a hard surface. If you're feeling a little down, that's no surprise. You're having a very normal response.

Having a normal response doesn't mean you have to suffer from depression. Plenty of help is out there for you. Start by talking to your physician or a mental health therapist. Online self-assessment tools can be really helpful. Two excellent sources for the tools along with resources you might find helpful are DepressionHurts. ca and MentalHealthAmerica.net. Please don't wait to find help.

I've found that just listening to my patients and encouraging them to talk about what they're feeling makes a big difference in their perception of their pain.

CHAPTER 15

CORTISONE INJECTIONS

C ortisone injections are the first go-to treatment for people whose plantar fasciitis is resistant to treatment. Cortisone is a synthetic hormone. It's similar to the hormone cortisol that your body produces in your adrenal glands, particularly when you're under stress. Among other roles, cortisol is your body's natural anti-inflammatory hormone.

When cortisone is injected into an inflamed area of the body, such as the plantar fascia, it acts as a local anti-inflammatory. For some people, this is just what they need to finally get out of pain. For others, however, the injections have no benefit. Unfortunately, we can't predict in advance who will respond and who won't. We can say that if the first cortisone injection doesn't work, there's little chance that a second one will.

CORTISONE CONS

Cortisone injections can be very helpful, but they do have some significant drawbacks. One potential problem is that the more cortisone injections you get over time, the greater your risk of rupturing your plantar fascia down the line (Lee et al. 2014). You get relief from the shots within a few days, but down the road, you could wind up with more foot problems. It's been suggested that up to 10 percent of patients who recover after a cortisone injection will later have a rupture in the plantar fascia.

An even bigger drawback to cortisone shots is that they're painful. A needle into your foot hurts.

If you have diabetes, a cortisone shot could significantly raise your blood sugar temporarily. Be sure to discuss this with your doctor before you decide to have the injection.

One of the possible side effects of a cortisone injection is a temporary flare of symptoms, including redness, heat, and an increase in pain. This may occur within twenty-four hours of the injection and should resolve somewhere within one to two days. Cold compresses can help relieve the symptoms. A flare of symptoms can be confused with redness, heat, and an increase in pain and swelling from an infection.

Infection often takes a few days to develop, though. If you recently had an injection and you experienced flare symptoms, go back to your doctor, podiatrist, or chiropodist and get checked. Nerve injury and even abscess formation at the injection site, although extremely rare, have been reported (Buccilli et al. 2005; Snow et al. 2005).

Another side effect of cortisone is a temporary softening of the tissues that come in contact with the drug itself. This can lead to tears of these tissues even with normal activity. Discuss precautions with your doctor before you go ahead with the injection. Cortisone injections shouldn't be attempted too frequently, as the cumulative effects can result in permanent weakening of the surrounding tissues.

A final con to cortisone injections is that the relief from the drug could be masking a mechanical problem. The shot will make you feel better for a couple of weeks, but then your problems are going to come back. I usually recommend taking care of the underlying biomechanical issues first. Only if your plantar fasciitis isn't responding or isn't responding enough would I suggest going on to the injection.

Because of the possible side effects and complications, cortisone should be used sparingly and not as a first-line option. We don't have any universal guidelines for cortisone shots, but most doctors recommend waiting at least four months between injections and not exceeding more than three injections for a total body area. Research published in the *Journal of Clinical Ultrasound* suggests that an ultrasound-guided injection is more precise and effective for injecting cortisone into plantar fasciitis. This may not be available, however. It may not be necessary, though, as most physicians are trained to inject the plantar fascia without ultrasound guidance. An additional risk of cortisone injections is that they may thin the fat pad under the heel. Ultrasound guidance lowers the risk that the injection will end up going into the fat pad, which cuts the chances for that particular complication.

PLATELET RICH PLASMA

Platelet rich plasma (PRP) is an injection that uses your own blood. Your platelets are tiny cell fragments that are a critical component in clotting and injury healing. Platelets are naturally extremely rich in connective tissue growth and healing factors. Studies suggest that the growth factors released by platelets recruit the body's natural repair cells to the area and help enhance the healing of muscles, tendons, and ligaments (Hsiao 2015).

To prepare the PRP injection, a small amount of your blood is removed and spun in a centrifuge. The platelets are spun out and concentrated to the point of being at above normal values. They're then injected into the plantar fascia where it originates in the heel.

The research so far suggests that a PRP shot seems to work about as well as a cortisone shot. Because PRP isn't a steroid hormone, however, it doesn't have the risk factors that go with cortisone injections. As with cortisone, the underlying mechanical issues still need to be addressed.

Platelet rich plasma is made from your own blood, so you don't have any risk of an allergic reaction or a drug interaction. It also doesn't soften tissues, so the risk of rupture is low when compared to cortisone.

A 2015 meta-analysis (a study of studies) published in the *Journal of Rheumatology* included seven trials. The researchers concluded that for the treatment of plantar fasciitis that has become resistant to treatment, PRP at three months was more effective than cortisone at lowering pain (Hsiao 2015). Shock wave therapy (to be discussed in the next chapter) and PRP provided similar pain relief at six months. The authors suggested that cortisone was the least effective at both the three- and six-month marks. They also suggested that while shock wave therapy was the least effective treatment at three months, at six months it lowered pain the most. So, in the short term, PRP may be better than cortisone, but for better long-term results, shock wave therapy may be more effective than both of them at six months (Hsiao 2015).

WHICH TO CHOOSE?

The effects of a cortisone shot are relatively short-lived, usually just a few months or less. Because it's an anti-inflammatory, cortisone will help to settle things down if your plantar fasciitis is inflammatory. If it's chronic and it's caused more by degeneration than inflammation, then the shot might not have any effect. If you've had plantar fasciitis for more than seven months, it may be degenerative. You might want to try a PRP shot instead, because platelet rich plasma doesn't do much for inflammation but is helpful for re-healing and growing new blood vessels to bring more blood flow to that area.

Cortisone is also the least expensive option. It's followed by PRP, which is significantly more expensive than cortisone—up to fifteen times more! Shock wave therapy can cost between $500 to $1,500.

CHAPTER 16

SHOCK WAVE THERAPY

S hock wave therapy is a noninvasive treatment for plantar fasciitis that uses pulses of high-energy acoustic waves, also called shock waves. The shock waves are delivered to the plantar fascia area as a way to relieve pain. The treatment began several decades ago as a way to break up kidney stones so they could pass easily. Since then, shock wave therapy has been developed as a way to treat tendon and fascia problems. Today, it's used to treat everything from plantar fasciitis to calcific shoulder tendinitis to rotator cuff problems to Achilles tendinitis. Recently, shock wave therapy has been noted to have an effect even in such things as wound healing in chronic diabetic foot ulcers.

How does shock wave therapy work? I don't know for sure. In fact, nobody can really say why it works. (Are you detecting a pattern here?) The mechanism of action for shock wave therapy is still largely unknown. Two theories might explain why it can be helpful for plantar fasciitis. One is that the pain of plantar fasciitis is thought to be reduced when the shock waves damage local cell membranes, which interferes with the transmission of pain signals. Another plausible theory is the shock waves increase the local blood flow to the plantar fascia and the surrounding area. Those areas are poorly vascularized to begin with, and now they are degenerated to the point where blood flow is even less. It's possible that the shock waves promote the growth of new blood vessels. Even if this happens at the microstructural level, it can bring more blood circulation to the area, which can certainly help with healing the affected tissues. At the end of the day, the intention is to make your PF a little bit worse to help promote healing that will start to make it better.

TYPES OF SHOCK WAVE THERAPY

Shock wave therapy essentially comes in two different types: high-dose and low-dose. High-dose therapy, as you would imagine, means a stronger, much more targeted, harder shock wave going into the soft tissues. It can be painful. Low-dose therapy typically is less painful but still sends the shock wave into the soft tissue. Today, most practitioners seem to prefer the low-dose approach. It seems to be about as effective as the high-dose treatment, but it's more comfortable for the patient. In my experience, patients don't feel pain from the treatment and are able to return to their everyday activities right away. Recent research suggests that six months after shock wave therapy, the reduction in pain is about equivalent to that from PRP therapy (Hsiao 2015).

The problem with any kind of shock wave therapy is that it takes at least three months before you start feeling any reduction in pain.

It takes that long for the plantar fascia to start to rebuild itself and repair the degeneration. In the meantime, patients should still continue all the other REST steps and wear their orthotics.

SAFETY AND SIDE EFFECTS

Shock wave therapy is pretty safe. Studies show that up to 40 percent of people who do high-dose therapy will have some superficial bruising on their skin. Other studies show about 70 percent of people who do any type of shock wave therapy will have redness of the skin where the shock wave was applied (Dizon et al. 2013). Overall, however, studies show that shock wave therapy doesn't really have any substantial side effects or complications.

A systematic review of shock wave therapy, published in the *British Journal of Sports Medicine* in 2014, looked at the effects of both high- and low-dose shock wave therapy for a number of tissue conditions, including plantar fasciitis. The researchers concluded that there was high-level evidence for both high and low-dose shock wave therapy as an effective treatment in chronic, nonresponding plantar fasciitis (Speed 2014).

Pain levels in patients treated with shock waves were reduced up to 72 percent, compared to only 44 percent in a placebo-controlled trial (Speed 2014). This fits with previous review research dating as far back as 2002, which suggested that shock wave therapy for patients with chronic plantar fasciitis had a success rate of up to 88 percent (Ogden 2002).

Both of these studies show that when direct shock waves are applied to the origin point of the plantar fascia on the under part of the heel, it's a safe and effective, nonsurgical method for treating chronic plantar fasciitis that's not responding to other treatment. It also suggests that shock wave therapy should be considered before surgical intervention and that it may be preferable to the known risks of cortisone injections.

PROS AND CONS

On the pro side, shock wave therapy is safe, with little in the way of side effects or complications. It's also fast. For low-dose shock wave therapy, I give my patients three treatments of seven minutes per foot, spaced out a week apart. Research and my own experience tell us that in cases that are resistant to treatment, up to two-thirds of people will respond well to shock wave therapy. Their pain will go down and their function will increase. Because it's pretty painless, some patients try shock wave therapy as an alternative to cortisone injections.

On the con side, low-dose shock wave therapy can cause mild discomfort at the application site; high-dose therapy can cause moderate pain at the application site. Shock wave therapy is expensive. In Canada, the cost can be anywhere between $600 and $800 per affected foot. If you have recalcitrant plantar fasciitis in both feet, the treatment could cost you $1,600 dollars—and sometimes insurance doesn't cover it. You might also be in the 33 percent of people who don't respond to the therapy. And then there's the twelve-week or longer wait to see if the treatment has helped you. If you're continuing all your other therapies at the same time and you finally start to get better, you can't really be sure that it was the shock treatment that did it.

When you're doing a lot of different things at once, it's hard to nail down which one thing is making the difference. But if you're five months into your plantar fasciitis treatment and you've seen no change despite doing the REST protocol and everything else, and then you do shock wave therapy and start to feel better, maybe the therapy really did help. Or maybe everything else you're doing is finally working—or as sometimes happens, your PF may have just spontaneously resolved on its own.

GETTING SHOCK WAVE TREATMENT

Getting shock wave treatment is pretty simple. You come into the office, remove your shoes and socks, and lie down on a treatment table. I apply ultrasound gel to your heel (it's clear, odorless, and washes off easily with water) and then use an applicator wand to send the shock waves into your heel. It sounds like a little hammer is tapping very loudly on your heel.

CHAPTER 17

SURGERY

If you're reading this part of the book, it's probably because you're still in a great deal of pain. Check back to page 179, where I talk about living with chronic pain. If you feel you can't live with the discomfort any longer, surgery may be an option for you.

I'm not a surgeon, so instead, I asked Ian Alexander, MD, a renowned orthopedic surgeon at Ohio State University's Wexner Medical Center, for his advice. He's the author of the classic text, *The Foot: Examination & Diagnosis* (Alexander 1997).

According to Dr. Alexander, "Surgery is rarely indicated for plantar fasciitis. The first-line therapy involves a stretching program and some kind of cushioning device in the shoe." He went on to say, "Usually, surgical intervention is not particularly effective. We try to avoid it unless we're out of options." He feels that custom-made foot orthotics can be a very effective treatment for plantar fasciitis. Not surprisingly for a leading foot surgeon, Dr. Alexander's comments are in line with what the current research says about surgery for plantar fasciitis.

Within the literature, there's a lot of debate about PF surgery, both about its value for reducing pain and about biomechanical outcomes related to surgery. The surgery usually involves cutting part of the plantar fascia. Some cadaver research has shown that when you surgically release even part of the plantar fascia, support for the arch is lost by up to 25 percent. For people with preexisting flat feet, release would only worsen their foot function. As most of this research is cadaver-based, however, we don't really know what all the consequences of surgical release are.

In living humans, some studies have reported no complications, while others report pain in the heel, top of the foot, scar tissue discomfort, and chronic pain after surgery. The duration and intensity of preoperative pain may affect the outcome. Patients who have been in pain longer may have worse results.

A retrospective analysis (looking back at patient records) that appeared in 2016 in *Foot & Ankle International* looked at a ten-year history of patients who had undergone an open release of their plantar fascia (MacInnes et al. 2016). Surveys were sent to the patients asking them about their foot pain an average of eighty months after their surgery. Based on the responses, the authors concluded that open release of the plantar fascia was of questionable clinical value (MacInnes et al. 2016). Patients may improve despite surgery simply as part of the natural course of plantar fasciitis.

In contrast, another retrospective analysis in the *Orthopaedic Journal of Sports Medicine* looked at follow-up surveys over a fifteen-year period; the average was seven years (Wheeler et al. 2014). The researchers found that 84 percent of respondents reported overall satisfaction with surgery; 16 percent were neutral or dissatisfied (Wheeler et al. 2014). In this study, 50 percent of cases were pain free; the mean pain improvement after surgery was 79 percent.

Both studies concluded that more research is needed to fully understand the short-, medium-, and long-term outcomes, both from a pain and biomechanical perspective.

While surgery may be an option for plantar fasciitis that has become resistant to treatment, I stress that all other conservative options should be considered and tried before consulting with a surgeon. Given the conflicting studies and overall lack of good information on outcomes, surgery should be considered only when all else has failed.

CHAPTER 18

WORK ACCOMMODATIONS

T he law in Canada says that employers have a duty to accommodate you if you need help to keep working with plantar fasciitis.
This is a complicated issue that's beyond my scope as a pedorthist.
Because it's so important, I've asked my friend Scott Matthews,
specialist II at Return to Work Services in the human resources
department of the city of London, to explain it.

THE DUTY TO ACCOMMODATE

What does the duty to accommodate mean? Employers have a
duty to accommodate employees with disabilities or injuries under
the Human Rights Code. Regardless of the size of the company, the employer, employee, and union (if there is one), all have
responsibilities to accommodate employees who qualify. They all
need to work together to ensure that the needs of all parties are
met. A large corporation has different stresses and opportunities
for accommodation than a smaller company, however.

An employer is not expect to accommodate an employee with a disability or injury by creating a job that doesn't exist or to offering work that is not meaningful or could be considered demeaning.

How can you work with your employer to ensure that a timely and safe return to transitional or permanently modified work is provided? The employee has some key ownership in initiating the process. With the assistance of the medical community, the employee is required to bring to the employer's attention the need for accommodation and the restrictions that the employer is to attempt to accommodate. In cases where the need is obvious, such as an employee who walks with crutches, the employer could be expected to initiate the conversation. Generally, however, it's up to employees to bring forward their accommodation needs with their appropriate workplace contact—usually their manager or someone in human resources, health services, or another relevant department.

As per the direction of the Canadian Medical Association, the employee's physician should provide the employer with any specific restrictions, along with the prognosis and the nature of the condition. Often, a collective agreement will ask for a physician to provide this information. However, most employers will accept and prefer restrictions provided by an appropriate treatment provider, such as a physiotherapist, occupational therapist, podiatrist, or chiropractor if the employee has physical accommodation needs.

To ensure that the information you provide your employer is helpful for creating accommodation for your difficulties, many employers have specific forms or letters. A standard treatment memo or functional abilities form or a custom letter assist the treating specialist in providing information that can be acted on. A note that simply says, "Off for medical reasons" doesn't help.

The specific diagnosis or treatment is confidential and can usually only be released to the employer with the permission of the employee. To make the accommodation, the employer needs information from the employee about restrictions, prognosis, and often the nature of a condition. Plantar fasciitis, for example, may require limited walking or standing for long periods while the individual participates in treatment. Even more helpful for making the accommodation is quantified information, such as "Standing and walking; five minutes, to be re-evaluated in two weeks." This type of information clearly assists your employer in proving an appropriate environment to allow you, as the employee, to take advantage of your treatment efforts. For example, if you work on an assembly line, the accommodation might be a stool that meets occupational health and safety standards so you don't have to stand.

If you need appliances to assist you in your recovery or on a permanent basis, review your coverage options with your benefit providers. There is no set plan of what is covered. Your internal benefit liaison may be able to advise you of your coverage levels and also inform you of what might be required to support a claim. If you do not have benefits, you may wish to discuss alternative treatments prior to investing in expensive appliances. For foot orthotics, many doctors recommend trying over-the-counter insoles before investing in custom orthotics.

POINTS TO REMEMBER

- Be prepared to help your employer help you by providing good information related to your job. Quantify it! Standing for five minutes each hour, or walking for ten minutes each hour, are clear directions that are hard to misinterpret. Your employer can use this information to screen jobs for you.

- Think about what "as tolerated" means to the employer in providing work and in their expectation of task completion. The more you own your part, the more likely your employer can help you.

- Have the requested restrictions presented as specifically as possible to avoid misinterpretation.

- Treatment memoranda or functional abilities forms are easy communication tools for both the health-care provider and the employer.

- Be as clear as possible about how long you may need accommodation.

- If your restriction is permanent and precludes you from performing the essential duties of your job, the Duty to Accommodate continues but the employer is not expected to create a new job for you.

- In some cases, temporarily "bundling" tasks can help. Say there are four building inspectors and one has a broken foot. Perhaps the inspector with the broken foot can do more of the administrative work while the others take on more of the fieldwork for a short time.

- Saturation is a consideration in accommodation. If only one of ten employees in a work group can do a task due to the others' restrictions, consideration is given as a result of saturation.

- Work on your personal health management plan and follow the directions of your treatment team. Limitations will impact you avocationally as well as vocationally.

DOCUMENTS FOR ACCOMMODATION

To help you provide the information your human resources department needs to accommodate you, I've posted some sample documents on my website at **thepfplan.com/hr**. You'll find research-based explanations and references about plantar fasciitis and why accommodation is needed to help you get better. I hope you never need to use this information, but many of my patients have found it very helpful.

PART FIVE

PREVENTION

INTRODUCTION TO PART FIVE

C ongratulations! If you're at this point in the book, your plantar fascia injury is feeling a lot better. You might even have recovered fully. Now it's time to do the things that can help keep you pain free and prevent a relapse. You want to reduce risk factors, strengthen your feet, and return to normal activity carefully.

CHAPTER 19

REDUCING RISK FACTORS

I discussed the risk factors for developing plantar fasciitis back in chapter 4. Some of the risk factors for getting plantar fasciitis are also risk factors for having it come back.

BODY MASS INDEX

The top risk factor for a relapse of your PF is having a high body mass index (BMI). If your BMI is 27 or greater, your risk of relapse is high. The normal range for BMI is 18 to 24, so 27 is in the overweight category. When you're taking ten thousand steps or more every day, those five, ten, fifteen or more extra pounds really add up.

Weight loss is never easy. I recommend getting professional help from experts on nutrition and lifestyle. PrecisionNutrition.com is an excellent starting point.

FLEXIBILITY

As we age, our range of motion naturally decreases. You can counteract that natural tendency by staying fit and doing things that help keep you flexible. This will really help reduce the likelihood of injury in the future.

Most of the elderly patients who come to see me because they have gait disturbances don't have other issues that affect the gait, such as Parkinson disease. Often their problems often come down to simple range of motion and flexibility loss. For example, loss of range of motion at the ankle can lead to decreased stability and increase the loads on both the plantar fascia and the Achilles tendon. Similarly, if your calf muscles aren't flexible enough to allow your leg to move over the top of your foot when you walk, your body compensates somewhere else. The easiest way to compensate for a gait disturbance is to pronate your foot (roll it in) or raise your heel prematurely. That puts even more strain on your plantar fascia.

Tight calf muscles and hamstrings can be risk factors for developing plantar fasciitis. To keep these muscles flexible, do the exercises in chapter 7 regularly. I've developed a complete lower leg flexibility program for preventing PF relapse. You can download it at **thepfplan.com/stretch**.

Yoga can be great for improving and maintaining general flexibility. Once you start to feel better, it's one of the best ways to improve and maintain your range of motion going forward. Be cautious at first about positions that put extra load on your feet, such as downward dog.

CONTINUE TO WEAR YOUR ORTHOTICS

I recommend continuing to wear your orthotics for at least six months after healing from your plantar fasciitis. Many of my patients find that once they're somewhere between 90 and 100 percent, their heel is still sensitive for at least six months afterward when they go barefoot. Keep wearing orthotics until that sensitivity goes away.

If you have a really high arch foot, that tends to put more pressure on the heel and the forefoot. That puts you at greater risk of developing plantar fasciitis to begin with and may put you at greater risk of relapse. Keeping your orthotics in can be a protective mechanism. If you have a really low arch, that can keep you from healing from your plantar fascia injury. I suggest wearing your orthotics for at least six months after you become pain free.

Once you're pain free for six months, talk to your specialist about tapering off your orthotics. I don't recommend just stopping. Not everyone can wean himself or herself off orthotics. If your plantar fasciitis was directly caused by faulty biomechanics and a decreased ability to handle cyclical soft tissue loading, you may need to continue with orthotics. If you do go off orthotics, get back into them the moment your pain starts to come back and then see your specialist to decide on the next steps.

HARD FLOORS AND BOOTS

Unless you change jobs, you probably won't be able to alter working on a hard floor. What you can change is your footwear. I talked about choosing the best shoes and boots back in chapter 9—shoes are the S in the REST protocol.

To prevent relapse, replace your work boots as soon as you start to see wear patterns that are more than half of the tread in one specific area. For instance, if the heel is really aggressively worn down but the other part of the boot looks brand-new, that wear pattern will start forcing you to walk in a way that will place odd stresses on your feet. You'll have to use the muscles of your feet and ankles more to stabilize your feet. That can also put extra strain on the plantar fascia and may cause a relapse.

Check the wear patterns of your shoes and boots regularly and get new footwear before it becomes an issue. Some of my patients need new boots every three months because of a combination of unforgiving floors and a few extra pounds.

If you're stuck with working on a hard floor, try to change positions often. Try to keep your lower limbs moving and avoid standing in one spot for extended periods of time. A good way to get your blood pumping and to relieve some of the stress on joints that have been in a static position for too long is to bend your knee and touch your heel to your butt. Sit whenever you can, even if it's just for a few minutes.

An often overlooked tip is to keep your work area clean and dry. Standing on a hard floor that's also slippery or dirty increases your risk of relapse. When you constantly have to balance yourself because the floor is slippery, you'll end up overworking the muscles in your feet and lower legs. You'll get fatigued quickly and put too much strain on your plantar fascia in order to maintain balance. This will fatigue you sooner and thus demand even more from your body after a full day at work.

PREGNANCY

If your feet and lower legs are swollen from pregnancy and you can no longer wear your usual shoes, or it's just uncomfortable to bend over and put shoes on, don't despair and go right for slippers or unsupported slip-ons. As I explained back in chapter 4, the average foot size change after pregnancy is anywhere between a half to one-and-a-half sizes. The hormones of pregnancy make your ligaments more prone to getting stretched out, plus you're now putting more weight on your foot. If you go barefoot a lot or wear shoes that don't fit well, your arch can collapse, which will widen and lengthen your foot. That makes you more prone to injuring the plantar fascia.

To reduce the discomfort of swelling, look into compression stockings. These help reduce swelling in your feet and legs so they don't get larger with time. Off-the-shelf and medical-grade stockings can be very effective. If you can't find these at your pharmacy, you can get them from a foot specialist or online. Sigvaris (sigvaris. com) and Sockwell (sockwell.us.com) make my favorite brands.

You don't have to be pregnant to have trouble bending down to put on your shoes. Instead of going barefoot or wearing loose slippers, go for slip-on shoes that don't skimp out on support. I recommend slip-ons that offer great arch support and cushioning. My favorite brands are New Balance 990 Slide, SOLE slide, SOLE flip-flop, and the Birkenstock Arizona. What I really hate to see are pregnant ladies who come in to see me wearing worn-out, slide-on sandals. These shoes are easy to get into and they're comfortable, but they're bad for your feet once they start to get past a certain point.

CHAPTER 20

FOOT STRENGTHENING

I f you've had plantar fasciitis once, you can get it again. If it does return, it may come back with a vengeance. While your first bout of plantar fasciitis may have responded to just six weeks of the REST protocol, your second bout could take as long as two years to heal completely. That's why prevention is crucial. Building up your foot strength is a really important part of preventing a relapse of plantar fasciitis. When the small muscles deep inside your foot are strong, the effects of fatigue will come on much later in the day. This will help keep your feet feeling great all day long and avoid strain on your plantar fascia.

I was fortunate to discuss foot strengthening with Dr. Irene S. Davis, PhD, PT, FAPTA, FACSM, FASB, director of the Spaulding National Running Center, Department of Physical Medicine and Rehabilitation, Harvard Medical School. Dr.

Davis shared her thinking about the role of orthotics and the value of exercise to strengthen the feet. She says,

> I do think there's a place to support the foot with orthotics in certain situations. I don't think orthotics are the Evil Empire. My overall sense, however, is that they're overused for musculoskeletal injuries. I actually think that in the acute phase, supporting the foot with an over-the-counter orthotic device or taping is a good idea. The foot is just like any other body part. If it's injured, you don't want to have it moving, so you splint it let it rest and heal. If someone has severe plantar fasciitis in the acute phase, the last thing you want to do is have them go without support.

I asked Dr. Davis what her advice would be for keeping plantar fasciitis from returning. She said,

> Keep the feet strong and flexible. I believe that you have small muscles in your feet that are stabilizers and not prime movers, just as you have muscles in your deep core that act in the same way. To have normal movement of the foot, I think you have to have a very stable foot core, just as you need a very stable lumbar core to prevent back pain. To have a stable, strong foot core, you need to focus on the intrinsic muscles, the ones that originate and insert in the foot. Of the intrinsic foot muscles, the ones to really focus on are the plantar muscles. You've got to do exercises that try to resist the deflection of your arch under load, because that's what strains the plantar fascia and gives it a repetitive load type injury.

What exercises does Dr. Davis recommend? She told me, "I think doming [also called arch lift or Janda's short foot] is probably one of the best exercises, because it works all the muscles that are underneath the foot. I recommend getting started with doming and other foot exercises as soon as you can do them without pain. Use your pain as a guide. Pain is your body's way of saying you know, this is too much load for me right now. It's a warning signal, a gift we're given. We use pain as a guide to customize treatment for each patient."

Dr. Davis points out,

> You can incorporate doming into your everyday activities, such as while you're standing in line at the grocery store checkout. We teach people how to do active standing, which starts with the foot but also includes some gluteus maximus and lower abdominal activation. It's amazing how different their posture looks when people start to do this. When I work with patients doing physical therapy for plantar fasciitis, we start with doming while sitting, then move on to doming while standing on two feet, then standing on one foot, then doming and hopping on two feet, then doming and hopping on one foot. It's a progression, just like any other exercise program, that moves from static to dynamic to more functional activities. I recommend doing your foot exercises ahead of an activity like running. The exercises activate the foot muscles and make you aware of them right from the start.

We discussed the question of why some people have a second bout of plantar fasciitis. Dr. Davis feels this is because doctors providing treatment at every level fail to emphasize or even think about foot strengthening. She says, "We think of the foot as a passive structure, so we don't think about strengthening it. I think one reason we have an epidemic of plantar fasciitis is that we're in supportive shoes all the time. In most cases, people probably don't need all that extra support. We're designed to go barefoot. When we wear minimal shoes without support or go barefoot, we strengthen the foot muscles. I think for treating PF we need to take the simplistic approach. Let the foot do what it was designed to do. In therapy, I give every foot a chance to be what it was naturally designed to be. By teaching our patients how to do foot exercises, we're able to wean almost all of them off their orthotics."

We also talked about the benefits of increasing foot strength beyond plantar fasciitis. She told me, "You avoid injuries to the foot. The majority of foot problems trace back to weak or imbalanced muscles. Foot exercises can help avoid bunions, stress fractures, and other problems." To find out more, please refer to the bibliography for the paper authored by McKeon et al., 2015.

FOOT STRENGTHENING EXERCISES

Start with one exercise, one set of ten reps. Once you're able to fully complete three full sets without pain or your foot cramping, then add in the next exercise. If you start all three at once, you run the risk of getting some seriously painful foot cramps.

The foot strengthening exercises I describe here aren't the same as the stretching exercises I talked about back in chapter 7. I suggest continuing with those exercises as a good way to stretch and maintain range of motion in your feet and ankles. Add these strengthening exercises once your foot pain is down to only 30 percent of what it was in the beginning.

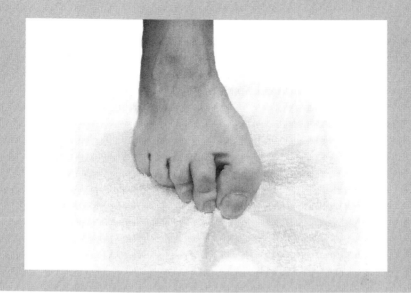

Towel Toe Curl

You need a small towel for this exercise.

- Put the towel on the floor.
- Sit in a chair and place your foot on the towel.
- Flex your toes hard enough to bunch up the towel.
- Hold for two seconds and then relax for five seconds.
- Repeat 10 times for each foot.

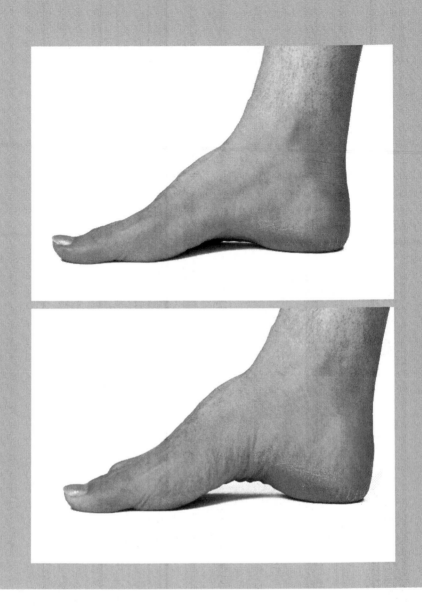

Arch Lift

This exercise is also called doming or Janda's short foot.

- Sit in a chair with your foot flat on the floor.
- Try to raise the arch of your foot by "scraping" the toes backward and contracting the muscles in the mid-back part of the arch.
- At the same time, keep the ball of your foot in contact with the floor. This may take some practice!
- Repeat 10 times for each foot.

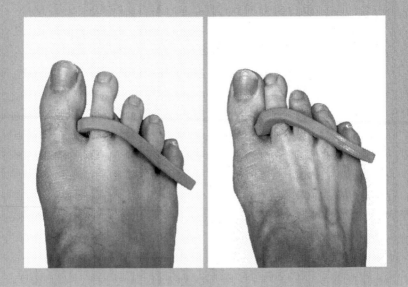

Toe Adduction

Adduction means pulling the toes together toward the centerline of your foot.

- Sit in a chair and place pedicure separators between your smaller toes. (You can get these at any pharmacy.)
- Pull your toes together. Hold for two seconds, push your toes apart, hold for two seconds and then relax for five seconds.
- To avoid cramping, start with just a few repetitions for each foot. Over a couple of weeks, work your way up to 10 repetitions for each foot.

CHAPTER 21

RETURNING TO ACTIVITY

W hen you take time off from activity to help your plantar fasciitis heal, your muscles atrophy, meaning they get weaker from disuse. For the smaller muscles, atrophy can start in as little as seventy-two hours; the larger muscles take longer. At the same time, you have a reduction in your cardiovascular fitness. Detraining of your cardiovascular fitness can happen in as little as ten days; significant detraining happens in two to four weeks (Neufer 1989). That's why I advocate for staying as active as possible while you do the REST protocol. You want to mitigate the damage from these two destructive processes.

Even if you stay as active as you can during this time, some weakness and loss of baseline fitness is inevitable. Once your foot doesn't hurt anymore, you'll naturally want to resume your regular activities and get back into shape as soon as possible. That's great, but be cautious. One of the main reasons people end up back in my office after they've recovered from plantar fasciitis is doing too much, too soon, too fast. They try to get right back to what they were doing without a gradual return.

What's gradual? If you've been away from your training for less than a couple of weeks, begin with 30 percent less of what you think you can do, as long as you can do that without a recurrence of pain. If you do have pain, cut back more. Gradually increase that by 10 percent per week. Again, if you have foot pain, cut back and increase more gradually.

If you've removed exercises that have aggravated your plantar fasciitis, such as planks, lunges, calf raises, and so on, start adding one back per week. If you feel foot pain, cut back or remove the exercise again. Once you're sure that you can successfully return to that exercise, add in the others in subsequent weeks. This is also a great time to talk with your medical professional, whether that's a foot specialist, physiotherapist, or physician, so that you're at the lowest possible risk of re-injury.

Returning to activity is just as much about balancing your mental preparedness with your physical. Mismatch either and you're asking to get hurt. I often see that all someone wants to do is get back to normal activity, whether it's walking the dog or playing competitive basketball. If you push yourself too fast, you can wind up reinjuring yourself. That can set you all the way back to where you were when the plantar fasciitis first started. At that point, you're at risk for demotivation and all the other health-related quality of life issues, including depression.

If you're not completely confident that returning to exercise won't lead to heel pain, you may subconsciously slightly alter your gait or how you work out. That could mean you put more pressure on the unaffected side, which in turn could lead to a new injury or plantar fasciitis in the other foot. Progressing slowly back to your previous activity level will help to build your confidence, strength, and endurance safely.

If you're completely de-trained, get back into exercise with activities that aren't intensively weight bearing. You might want to use the elliptical machine at first instead of going straight back to Zumba class.

RETURNING TO RUNNING

Let's say you were running 5K five times a week. Start back at 3 to 3.5K total for a week or two; cut back if you have foot pain. If you don't have foot pain, increase your distance by 10 percent each week until you're back to your previous distance and frequency.

If you're completely de-trained because you've been away from running for more than four weeks, you might need to start back at a learn-to-run protocol. The idea of the protocol is to get you back to running your usual distance with the lowest likelihood of getting hurt.

• • •

LEARN TO RUN AGAIN

Week	Run	Walk	Reps	Total Work-out Time	Sessions Per Week	Rest Days Between Runs
1 to 4	1 min • Increase by 1 min per week	4 mins • Decrease by 1 min per week	3	15 mins	3	2
5 to 6	5 to 8 mins • Increase by 1 min per week	1 min • Walk 1 min after each running set	3 • At week 6, add one more set	18 to 27 mins	3	2
9 to 12	9 to 10 mins • Once you reach 10 mins of running, hold there	1 min	3	30 to 33 mins	3	2

The running protocol can feel painfully slow. It starts with just fifteen minutes: one minute of running and four minutes of walking, repeated three times with two days of rest in between. It's slow. It's designed to be that way, because if you've been struggling with plantar fasciitis for some time, the last thing you want is a new injury or, just as bad, PF in the other foot. You may feel like you're hardly exercising, but if you're completely de-trained, the next day you'll feel like you've been hit by a truck. The protocol slowly allows your muscles, tendons, ligaments, and bones to get used to the new loads and to fully recover before the next run.

Remember to listen to your body. If one day you're completely tired and can barely get in the mood for running, skip it. Get a great night's rest and go on to the next day. Consistency is important with exercise, but I don't think consistency at the risk of having a new injury is worth it.

REPLACE YOUR FOOTWEAR

Footwear is crucial for maintaining good foot health. Make sure that your shoes are replaced at regular intervals. Replacing your shoes every two years will just not suffice. Most shoes aren't built to last much more than eight to twelve months, especially if you're doing something active in them on consecutive days. The material deep inside the shoe doesn't have time to fully rebound or recover, so it wears out even faster.

The wear pattern on the sole of your shoe can tell you volumes about the condition of your footwear. It's literally where the rubber hits the road, as you can see from these pictures. If your athletic shoes are worn down completely within two to three months of

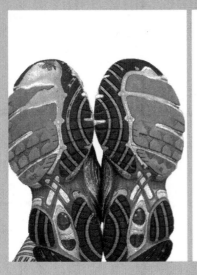
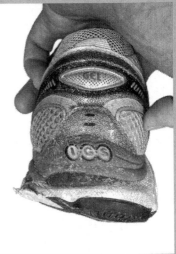

purchasing them and you're not running 100 kilometers a week, the fit of the shoe might be wrong or the shoe might not be properly matched to your foot type. I suggest talking to a qualified foot specialist or a salesperson at a specialty shoe store. They can both be great sources of information about getting the right fit for your foot. You can find more information about shoe selection on my website at **thepfplan.com/footwear.**

Running shoes should be replaced every 500 to 600 kilometers of total distance. If you run 50 kilometers a week and you're running overall 200 kilometers a month, then at the end of the day you're going to be replacing your shoes much faster than the 5K runner who might only do 20 kilometers a week. Some of my patients buy new shoes every three weeks because they run 200 kilometers a week. They're Olympic hopefuls, so they blow through shoes super-fast.

Steel-toed work boots should be replaced every six to eight months if you're wearing them all day every day. Look for the wear pattern in the tread. If you're standing on hard floors or in things that are particularly corrosive, certain oils for instance, your boots will break down much faster.

Casual shoes, the kind you wear to work, usually last for about a year. Check the wear pattern and replace them more often if needed.

YOU CAN BE PAIN FREE

H ere's what my patients with plantar fasciitis have told me over the years:

- It's hopeless.
- It will take months for me to get better.
- I need to stop all activity so my foot can heal.
- It'll go away on its own.
- Going barefoot will help.
- I need those expensive custom orthotics right now.

Now that you've read this book, you know that none of the afore-mentioned statements are true. The reality is that by following the REST protocol and the other information in this book, your plantar fasciitis can heal. *You can feel better tomorrow.*

How much better? If you're diligent with the REST protocol, it might only take six weeks to become pain free. Based on your individual situation, you might need longer to progress through Phases 2 or 3, but never give up. In my experience, plantar fasciitis can be treated successfully almost every time.

SUCCESS STORIES

I have treated thousands of people with plantar fasciitis. By the time they come to me, they've often been in pain for months—they're ready to just give up on ever returning to normal. I work with them to incorporate the REST protocol, examine or re-examine their need for orthotics of all types, and consider the possibility of more invasive forms of treatment. Treatment can sometimes be time-consuming and even a bit frustrating, but as my patient Morticia explains, healing your plantar fasciitis gives you back your life.

Morticia's Story

I am a fitness instructor, and I suffered with plantar fasciitis for almost two years, in spite of having tried physiotherapy. High-impact exercise left me limping and reaching for anti-inflammatories. My husband had previously had the same problem and had experienced great improvement after trying the services of a local pedorthist, Colin Dombroski, at SoleScience. I decided to see if Colin could help me. Along with fitting me for orthotics, he gave me exercises to strengthen the muscles in my feet and exercises to relieve the tension in my fascia so that they could heal while I still maintained my exercise regimen. That, together with the orthotics, literally changed my life. I was able to increase the intensity of my exercise and was once again

*confident in doing high-impact aerobics. As a nice side effect, I
lost a significant amount of weight! Just one week after starting to
wear the orthotics, I noticed immediate results, even when I wasn't
exercising. I was able to become pain free and greatly increase
my range of motion. I increased the impact and intensity of my
workouts and could walk long distances without feeling any pain or
stress in my feet. I appreciate that Colin is also an athlete and able
to identify with the unique range of needs presented by his patients.*

FOR MORE INFORMATION

My website at **thepfplan.com** is full of resources for people with
plantar fasciitis and for the health-care professionals who treat
them. The site has information about every aspect of managing,
treating, and preventing PF. I also have an online store to help
you find the right off-the-shelf orthotics and other devices, such
as night splints and compression socks.

The website has videos of me demonstrating the stretching and
strengthening exercises I recommend, videos of me interviewing
other specialists about plantar fasciitis treatment, and videos of
patient testimonials.

I've set up an online community so people with plantar fasciitis
can share information and experiences and get their questions
answered. To learn more about the group, please visit **thepfplan.
com/community**.

For health-care professionals, the website has links to important
research papers and information about my accredited continuing
education course.

I'm here to help. You can reach me at colin@thepfplan.com. I'd love to hear how this book helped you. If you're interested in having my team help you implement the stages of this book, please visit **thepfplan.com/yourteam** to find out how we can work with you one-on-one to personalize your treatment plan.

Leonardo da Vinci said, "The human foot is a masterpiece of engineering and a work of art." Let's work together to get you back on yours.

To your good health,

Colin

ACKNOWLEDGMENTS

A s the great Sir Winston Churchill said, "Writing a book is an adventure. To begin with, it is a toy and an amusement. Then it becomes a mistress, then it becomes a master, then it becomes a tyrant. The last phase is that just as you are about to be reconciled to your servitude, you kill the monster and fling him to the public."

Many people generously contributed their time, support, and guidance to me while I was writing this book. Of course, I'll try to be as inclusive as possible, but if I have left anyone out, it is by no means intentional. You know I love you!

I'd like to thank Dr. Tatiana Jevremovic for her kind words of support and kicks in the butt! Dr. Robert Litchfield for his generous foreword and unwavering support. Robert Ditchfield for being a sounding board when needed. To the entire team at SoleScience, thank you for your help and your patience as I went through this lengthy process.

A special thank you to Adam Froats and Megan Balsdon, who helped compile the research.

To those who had a chance to review the book and give feedback/praise, Dr. Frank Shin, Louise Karch, Domenic DiNardo, Christy Shantz, Brenda De Pauw, Theodore J. Madison, Robert Neill, Jim Cook, Rick Melo, Christine Rowe, and Susan McMurray, thank you for taking time out to help.

Thank you, Tucker, for your help in the beginning and providing the contacts to get this project off the ground. Thank you to the wonderful people at BIAB, with a special note going to Sheila. I enjoyed our talks so much that I'll have to start thinking about book two now!

To my contributors, Dr. Tatiana Jevremovic, April Crake, Dr. Irene Davis, Scott Mathews, Greg Alcock, and Dr. Ian Alexander, without your time and effort, this book would only be half of what it is today. Thank you for lending your expertise.

To Jayson Gaignard, Kandis Marie, and Joey Coleman, I can't begin to describe the way that weekend changed my life other than to say if it wasn't for IPO, this book wouldn't exist, and I wouldn't be the changed man, father, and entrepreneur I am today. A million times, thank you.

Another special thanks goes to the wonderful and talented Sara Stibitz for her help on crafting some of the marketing messages. Thanks also to the IPO group, Laurence Tham, Shane Stott, Anton Zolotov, Nicole Welch, Luke Harris-Gallahue, Randal

Wark, Craig Bongelli, Domenic DiNardo, Rikke Hansen, Davina Hearne, Darryl Hicks, James Perly, Christina West, Tahani Aburaneh, UJ Ramdas, Chris Plough, Ali Blye Abrahamy, Mathieu Lachaîne, Brent Thacker, Ryan Hawk, Kenton Ho, Neeley Koester, Reggie Chandra, Mark Fullerton, Sarah McBride Thacker, Tiffany Turner Cavegn, Christine Hanna Fullerton, and Garrett Gunderson. Thank you for the encouragement through the IPO experience. To those who chimed in here and there on the group chats, your input helped shape this book too! Rock on.

BIBLIOGRAPHY

Alexander, I. J. *The Foot: Examination & Diagnosis.* 2nd ed. London: Churchill Livingstone, 1997.

Alshami, A. M., T. Souvlis, and M. W. Coppieters. "A Review of Plantar Heel Pain of Neural Origin: Differential Diagnosis and Management." *Manual Therapy*, 13, no. 2 (2008): 103–111.

Alvarez-Nemegyei, J., and J. J. Canoso. "Heel Pain: Diagnosis and Treatment, Step By Step." *Cleveland Clinic Journal of Medicine*, 73, no. 5 (2006): 465–471.

American Academy of Family Physicians. "Plantar Fasciitis: What You Should Know." *American Family Physician*, 72, no. 11 (2005): 2247–2248.

Anderson, J., and J. Stanek. "Effect of Foot Orthoses as Treatment for Plantar Fasciitis or Heel Pain." *Journal of Sport Rehabilitation*, 22, no. 2 (2013): 130–136.

Attard, J., and D. Singh. "A Comparison of Two Night Ankle-Foot Orthoses Used in the Treatment of Inferior Heel Pain: A Preliminary Investigation." *Foot and Ankle Surgery*, 18, no. 2 (2012): 108–110.

Baldassin, V., C. R. Gomes, and P. S. Beraldo. "Effectiveness of Prefabricated and Customized Foot Orthoses Made From Low-Cost Foam for Noncomplicated Plantar Fasciitis: A Randomized Controlled Trial." *Archives of Physical Medicine and Rehabilitation*, 90, no. 4 (2009): 701–706.

Balsdon, M. E. R., K. M. Bushey, C. E. Dombroski, M.-E. Lebel, and T. R. Jenkyn. "Medial Longitudinal Arch Angle Presents Significant Differences Between Foot Types: A Biplane Fluoroscopy Study." *Journal of Biomechanical Engineering*, 138, no. 10 (2016): 101007.

Beardwood, B. A., B. Kirsh., and N. J. Clark. (2005). "Victims Twice Over: Perceptions and Experiences of Injured Workers." *Qualitative Health Research*, 15, no. 1 (2005): 30–48.

Beeson, P. "Plantar fasciopathy: Revisiting the risk factors." *Foot and Ankle Surgery*, 20, no. 3 (2014): 160–165.

Beischer, A. D., A. Clarke, R. N. de Steiger, L. Donnan, A. Ibuki, and R. Unglik. "The Practical Application of Multimedia Technology to Facilitate the Education and Treatment of Patients with Plantar Fasciitis: A Pilot Study." *Foot and Ankle Specialist*, 1, no. 1 (2008): 30–38.

"Body Composition of Adults, 2012 to 2013," Statistics Canada, accessed September 30, 2016, http://www.statcan.gc.ca/pub/82-625-x/2014001/article/14104-eng.htm.

Bolívar, Y. A., P. V. Munuera, and J. P. Padillo. "Relationship between Tightness of the Posterior Muscles of the Lower Limb and Plantar Fasciitis." *Foot & Ankle International*, 34, no. 1 (2013): 42–48.

Buccilli Jr., T. A., H. R. Hall, and J. D. Solmen. "Sterile Abscess Formation Following a Corticosteroid Injection for the Treatment of Plantar Fasciitis." *Journal of Foot and Ankle Surgery*, 44, no. 6 (2005): 466–468.

Burns, J., K. B. Landorf, M. Ryan, J. Crosbie, and R. Ouvrier. "Interventions for the Prevention and Treatment of Pes Cavus (High-Arched Foot Deformity)." *Cochrane Database Systematic Reviews*, Issue 4 (2007): 8–10.

Chang, R., P. A. Rodrigues, Van Emmerik, and J. Hamill. "Multi-Segment Foot Kinematics and Ground Reaction Forces during Gait of Individuals with Plantar Fasciitis." *Journal of Biomechanics*, 47, no. 11 (2014): 2571–2577.

Chevalier, T. L., and N. Chockalingam. "Effects of Foot Orthoses: How Important Is the Practitioner?" *Gait and Posture*, 35, no. 3 (2012): 383–388.

Chia, J. K. K., M. Aust, S. Suresh, D. B. Eng, A. Kuah, D. B. Eng, ... D. B. Eng. "Comparative Trial of the Foot Pressure Patterns between Corrective Orthotics, Formthotics , Bone Spur Pads and Flat Insoles in Patients with Chronic Plantar Fasciitis." *Annals of Academy of Medicine Singapore*, 38, no. 10 (2009): 869–875.

Chundru, U., A. Liebeskind, F. Seidelmann, J. Fogel, P. Franklin, and J. Beltran, J. "Plantar Fasciitis and Calcaneal Spur Formation Are Associated with Abductor Digiti Minimi Atrophy on MRI of the Foot." *Skeletal Radiology*, 37, no. 6 (2008): 505–510.

Cole, C., C. Seto, and J. Gazewood. "Plantar Fasciitis: Evidence-Based Review of diagnosis and Therapy." *American Family Physician*, 72, no. 11 (2005): 2237–2242.

Cornwall, M. W., and T. G. McPoil. "Plantar Fasciitis: Etiology and Treatment." *Journal of Orthopaedic & Sports Physical Therapy*, 29, no. 12 (1999): 756–760.

Cotchett, M. P., S. Munteanu, and K. B. Landorf. "Depression, Anxiety, and Stress in People with and without Plantar Heel Pain." *Foot & Ankle International*, 37, no. 8 (2016): 816–821.

Coyle, E. F., M. K. Hemmert, and A. R. Coggan. "Effects of Detraining on Cardiovascular Responses to Exercise: Role of Blood Volume." *Journal of Applied Physiology*, 60, no. 1 (1986): 95–99.

Cutts, S., N. Obi, C. Pasapula, and W. Chan. "Plantar Fasciitis." *Annals of the Royal College of Surgeons of England*, 94, no. 8 (2012): 539–542.

DiGiovanni, B. F., D. A. Nawoczenski, M. E. Lintal, E. A. Moore, J. C. Murray, G. E. Wilding, and J. F. Baumhauer. "Tissue-Specific Plantar Fascia-Stretching Exercise Enhances Outcomes in Patients with Chronic Heel Pain." *Journal of Bone and Joint Surgery*, 85-A, no. 7 (2003): 1270–1277.

Dizon, J. N., C. Gonzalez-Suarez, M. T. Zamora, and E. D. Gambito. "Effectiveness of Extracorporeal Shock Wave Therapy in Chronic Plantar Fasciitis: A Meta-Analysis." *American Journal of Physical Medicine & Rehabilitation*, 92, no. 7 (2013): 606–620.

Drake, M., C. Bittenbender, and R. E. Boyles. "The Short-Term Effects of Treating Plantar Fasciitis with a Temporary Custom Foot Orthosis and Stretching." *Journal of Orthopaedic and Sports Physical Therapy*, 41, no. 4 (2011): 221–231.

Eng, J. J., and M. R. Pierrynowski. "The Effect of Soft Foot Orthotics on Three-Dimensional Lower-Limb Kinematics during Walking and Running." *Physical Therapy*, 74, no. 9 (1994): 836–844.

Ferber, R., and B. Benson. "Changes in Multi-Segment Foot Biomechanics with a Heat-Mouldable Semi-Custom Foot Orthotic Device." *Journal of Foot and Ankle Research*, 4, no. 1 (2011): 18–25.

Ferber, R., and B. Hettinga. "A Comparison of Different Over-the-Counter Foot Orthotic Devices on Multi-Segment Foot Biomechanics." *Prosthetics and Orthotics International*, (2015): 1–7.

Fong, D. T. P., K. Y. Pang, M. M. L. Chung, A. S. L. Hung, and K. M. Chan. "Evaluation of Combined Prescription of Rocker Sole Shoes and Custom-Made Foot Orthoses for the Treatment of Plantar Fasciitis." *Clinical Biomechanics*, 27, no. 10 (2012): 1072–1077.

Fryar, C., M. Carroll, and C. Ogden. "Prevalence of overweight, obesity, and extreme obesity among adults: United States, trends 1960–1962 through 2009–2010." Atlanta, GA: *National Center of Health Statistics* (2012).

Gatchel, R. J. "Comorbidity of Chronic Pain and Mental Health Disorders : The Biopsychosocial Perspective." *American Psychologist*, 59, no. 8 (November 2004): 731–738.

Genc, H., M. Saracoglu, B. Nacir, H. R. Erdem, and M. Kacar. "Long-Term Ultrasonographic Follow-Up of Plantar Fasciitis Patients Treated with Steroid Injection." *Joint Bone Spine*, 72, no. 1 (2005): 61–65.

Goff, J. D., and R. Crawford. "Diagnosis and Treatment of Plantar Fasciitis." *American Family Physician*, 84, no. 6 (2011): 676–682.

Gross, M. T., J. M. Byers, J. L. Krafft, Lackey, and Melton. "The Impact of Custom Semirigid Foot Orthotics on Pain and Disability for Individuals with Plantar Fasciitis." *Journal of Orthopaedic and Sports Physical Therapy*, 32, no. 4 (2002): 149–157.

Gu, Y. D., Li, Lake, Zeng, Ren, and Li. "Image-Based Midsole Insert Design and the Material Effects on Heel Plantar Pressure Distribution during Simulated Walking Loads." *Computer Methods in Biomechanics and Biomedical Engineering*, 14, no. 8 (2011): 747–753.

Harty, J., K. Soffe, G. O'Toole, and Stephens. "The Role of Hamstring Tightness in Plantar Fasciitis." *Foot & Ankle International*, 26, no. 12 (2005): 1089–1092.

Hawke, F., J. Burns, J. Radford, and V. du Toit. "Custom-Made Foot Orthoses for the Treatment of Foot Pain (Review)." *Cochrane Collaboration*, no. 3 (2008): 1–20.

Hohmann, E., P. Reaburn, and A. Imhoff. "Runner's Knowledge of Their Foot Type: Do They Really Know?" The *Foot*, 22, no. 3 (2012): 205–210.

Hsiao, M. Y., C. Y. Hung, K. V. Chang, K. L. Chien, and Y. K. Wang. "Comparative Effectiveness of Autologous Blood-Derived Products, Shock-Wave Therapy and Corticosteroids for Treatment of Plantar Fasciitis: A Network Meta-Analysis." *Rheumatology*, 54, no. 9 (2015): 1735–1743.

Hsu, Y. C., Gung, Shih, C. K. Feng, S. H. Wei, C. H. Yu, and C. S. Chen. "Using an Optimization Approach to Design an Insole for Lowering Plantar Fascia Stress— A Finite Element Study." *Annals of Biomedical Engineering*, 36, no. 8 (2008): 1345–1352.

Huang, C. K. "Biomechanical Evaluation of Longitudinal Arch Stability." *Foot & Ankle*, 14, no. 6 (1993): 353.

Irving, D. B., J. L. Cook, and H. B. Menz. "Factors Associated with Chronic Plantar Heel Pain: A Systematic Review." *Journal of Science and Medicine in Sport*, 9, no. 1–2 (2006): 11–22.

Irving, D. B., J. L. Cook, M. A. Young, and H. B. Menz. "Obesity and Pronated Foot Type May Increase the Risk of Chronic Plantar Heel Pain: A Matched Case-Control Study." *BMC Musculoskeletal Disorders*, 8, no. 1, (2007): 41-48.

———. "Impact of Chronic Plantar Heel Pain on Health-Related Quality of Life." *Journal of the American Podiatric Medical Association*, 98, no. 4 (2008): 283–289.

Kim, C., M. R. Cashdollar, R. W. Mendicino, A. R. Catanzariti, L. Fuge, L. "Incidence of Plantar Fascia Ruptures Following Corticosteroid Injection." *Foot & Ankle Specialist*, 3, no. 6 (2010): 335–337.

Kirby, K. A. "Understanding Ten Key Biomechanical Functions of the Plantar Fascia." *Podiatry Today*, 29, no. 7 (2016): 1–12.

Kirsh, B., T. Slack and C. A. King. "The Nature and Impact of Stigma Towards Injured Workers." *Journal of Occupational Rehabilitation*, 22, no. 1 (2012): 143–154.

Knapik, J. J., D. W. Trone, J. Tchandja, and B. H. Jones. "Injury-Reduction Effectiveness of Prescribing Running Shoes on the Basis of Foot Arch Height: Summary of Military Investigations." *Journal of Orthopaedic & Sports Physical Therapy*, 44, no. 10 (2014): 805–812.

Landorf, K. B. "Orthotics Not Effective for Plantar Fasciitis." *Journal of Family Practice*, 55, no. 10 (2006): 1305–1310.

Landorf, K. B., A.-M. Keenan, and R. D. Herbert. "Effectiveness of Foot Orthoses to Treat Plantar Fasciitis: A Randomized Trial." *Archives of Internal Medicine*, 166, no. 12 (2006): 1305–1310.

————. "Customized or Prefabricated Foot Orthoses Improved Function Only in the Short Term in Patients with Plantar Fasciitis." *Journal of Bone and Joint Surgery*, 89-A, no. 2 (2007): 458.

Landorf, K. B., and H. B. Menz. "Plantar Heel Pain and Fasciitis." *Clinical Evidence*, 2, no. 1111 (2008): 1–18.

Lee, H. S., Y. R. Choi, S. W. Kim, J. Y. Lee, J. H. Seo, and J. J. Jeong. "Risk Factors Affecting Chronic Rupture of the Plantar Fascia." *Foot & Ankle International*, 35, no. 3 (2014): 258–263.

Lee, S. Y., P. McKeon, and J. Hertel. "Does the Use of Orthoses Improve Self-Reported Pain and Function Measures in Patients with Plantar Fasciitis? A Meta-Analysis." *Physical Therapy in Sport*, 10, no. 1 (2009): 12–18.

Lee, T. G., and T. S. Ahmad. "Intralesional Autologous Blood Injection Compared to Corticosteroid Injection for Treatment Of Chronic Plantar Fasciitis. A Prospective, Randomized, Controlled Trial." *Foot & Ankle International*, 28, no. 9 (2007): 984–990.

Lee, W. C. C., W. Y. Wong, E. Kung, and A. K. L. Leung. "Effectiveness of Adjustable Dorsiflexion Night Splint in Combination with Accommodative Foot Orthosis on Plantar Fasciitis." *Journal of Rehabilitation Research and Development*, 49, no. 10 (2012): 1557–1564.

Lee, W. E. "An Historical Appraisal and Discussion of the Root Model as a Clinical System of Approach in the Present Context of Theoretical Uncertainty." *Clinics in Podiatric Medicine and Surgery*, 18, no. 4 (2001): 555–684.

Lewis, R. D., P. Wright, and L. H. McCarthy. "Orthotics Compared to Conventional Therapy and Other Non-Surgical Treatments for Plantar Fasciitis." *Journal of the Oklahoma State Medical Association*, 108, no. 12 (2015): 596–598.

Li, Z., T. Jin, and Z. Shao. "Meta-Analysis of High-Energy Extracorporeal Shock Wave Therapy in Recalcitrant Plantar Fasciitis." *European Journal of Medical Sciences: Swiss Medical Weekly*, 143, (2013): w13825.

MacInnes, A., S. C. Roberts, J. Kimpton, and A. Pillai. "Long-Term Outcome of Open Plantar Fascia Release." *Foot & Ankle International*, 37, no. 1 (2016): 17–23.

Malisoux, L., N. Chambon, N. Delattre, N. Gueguen, A. Urhausen, and D. Theisen. "Injury Risk in Runners Using Standard or Motion-Control Shoes: A Randomised Controlled Trial with Participant and Assessor Blinding." *British Journal of Sports Medicine*, 50, no. 8 (2016): 481–487.

Martin, R. L., T. E. Davenport, S. F. Reischl, T. G. McPoil, J. W. Matheson, D. K. Wukich, ... J. J. Godges. "Heel Pain—Plantar Fasciitis: Revision 2014." *Journal of Orthopaedic & Sports Physical Therapy*, 44, no. 11 (2014): A1–A33.

Mckeon, P. O., J. Hertel, D. Bramble, and I. Davis. "The Foot Core System: A New Paradigm for Understanding Intrinsic Foot Muscle Function." *British Journal of Sports Medicine*, 49, no. 290 (2014): 290–298.

McPoil, T. G., and G. C. Hunt. Evaluation and Management of Foot and Ankle Disorders: Present Problems and Future Directions. *Journal of Orthopaedic and Sports Physical Therapy*, 21, no. 6 (1995): 381–388.

Merskey, H., and N. Bogduk, eds. *Classification of Chronic Pain. Descriptions of Chronic Pain Syndromes and Definitions of Pain Terms*. 2nd ed. Seattle: International Association for the Study of Pain, 2002.

Michelsson, O., Y. T. Konttinen, P. Paavolainen, and S. Santavirta. "Plantar Heel Pain and Its 3-Mode 4-Stage Treatment." *Modern Rheumatology*, 15, no. 5 (2005): 307–314.

Miller, J. E., B. M. Nigg, W. Liu, D. J. Stefanyshyn, and M. A. Nurse. "Influence of Foot, Leg and Shoe Characteristics on Subjective Comfort." *Foot & Ankle International*, 21, no. 9 (2000): 759–767.

Mills, K., P. Blanch, and B. Vicenzino. "Influence of Contouring and Hardness of Foot Orthoses on Ratings of Perceived Comfort." *Medicine and Science in Sports and Exercise*, 43, no. 8 (2011): 1507–1512.

———. "Comfort and Midfoot Mobility Rather Than Orthosis Hardness or Contouring Influence Their Immediate Effects on Lower-Limb Function in Patients with Anterior Knee Pain." *Clinical Biomechanics*, 27, no. 1 (2012): 202–208.

Mujika, I., and S. Padilla. "Detraining: Loss of Training-Induced Physiological and Performance Adaptations. Part I." *Sports Medicine*, 30, no. 2 (2000): 79–87.

———. "Detraining: Loss of Training-Induced Physiological and Performance Adaptations. Part II: Long-Term Insufficient Training Stimulus." *Sports Medicine*, 30, no. 3 (2000): 145–154.

Mündermann, A., B. M. Nigg, R. N. Humble, and D. J. Stefanyshyn. "Orthotic Comfort Is Related to Kinematics, Kinetics, and EMG in Recreational Runners." *Medicine and Science in Sports and Exercise*, 35, no. 10 (2003): 1710–1719.

Mündermann, A., B. M. Nigg, D. J. Stefanyshyn, and R. N. Humble. "Development of a Reliable Method to Assess Footwear Comfort during Running." *Gait and Posture*, 16, no. 1 (2002): 38–45.

Mündermann, A., D. J. Stefanyshyn, and B. M. Nigg. "Relationship between Footwear Comfort of Shoe Inserts and Anthropometric and Sensory Factors." *Medicine and Science in Sports and Exercise*, 33, no. 11 (2001): 1939–1945.

Neufer, P. D. "The Effect of Detraining and Reduced Training on the Physiological Adaptations to Aerobic Exercise Training." *Sports Medicine*, 8, no. 5 (1989): 302–320.

Ogden, J. A., R. G. Alvarez, and M. Marlow. "Shockwave Therapy for Chronic Proximal Plantar Fasciitis: A Meta-Analysis." *Foot & Ankle International*, 23, no. 4 (2002): 301–308.

Oliveira, H. A. V., A. Jones, E. Moreira, F. Jennings, and J. Natour. "Effectiveness of Total Contact Insoles in Patients with Plantar Fasciitis." *Journal of Rheumatology*, 42, no. 5 (2015): 870–878.

Ontario Human Rights Commission. *Policy and Guidelines on Disability and the Duty to Accommodate* (2009).

Orchard, J. "Plantar Fasciitis." *British Medical Journal*, 345 (2012): e6603.

Osborne, H. R., W. H. Breidahl, and G. T. Allison. "Critical Differences in Lateral X-Rays with and without a Diagnosis of Plantar Fasciitis." *Journal of Science and Medicine in Sport*, 9, no. 3 (2006): 231–237.

Patel, A., and B. DiGiovanni. "Association between Plantar Fasciitis and Isolated Contracture of the Gastrocnemius." *Foot & Ankle International*, 32, no. 1 (2011): 5–8.

Pohl, M. B., J. Hamill, and I. S. Davis. "Biomechanical and Anatomic Factors Associated with a History of Plantar Fasciitis in Female Runners." *Clinical Journal of Sport Medicine*, 19, no. 5 (2009): 372–376.

Ribeiro, A. P., S. M. A. João, R. C. Dinato, V. D. Tessutti, and I. C. N. Sacco. "Dynamic Patterns of Forces and Loading Rate in Runners with Unilateral Plantar Fasciitis: A Cross-Sectional Study." *PLoS ONE*, 10, no. 9 (2015): 1–9.

Ribeiro, A. P., F. Trombini-Souza, V. D. Tessutti, F. R. Lima, S. M. João, and I. C. N. Sacco. "The Effects of Plantar Fasciitis and Pain on Plantar Pressure Distribution of Recreational Runners." *Clinical Biomechanics*, 26, no. 2 (2011): 194–199.

Ribeiro, A. P., F. Trombini-Souza, V. Tessutti, F. R. Lima, I. C. N. Sacco, S. João. "Rearfoot Alignment and Medial Longitudinal Arch Configurations of Runners with Symptoms and Histories of Plantar Fasciitis." *Clinics*, 66, no. 6 (2011): 1027–1033.

Riddle, D. L., M. Pulisic, and K. Sparrow. "Impact of Demographic and Impairment-Related Variables on Disability Associated with Plantar Fasciitis." *Foot & Ankle International*, 25, no. 5 (2004): 311–317.

Roos, E., M. Engström, and B. Söderberg. "Foot Orthoses for the Treatment of Plantar Fasciitis." *Foot & Ankle International*, 27, no. 8 (2006): 606–611.

Ross, M. "Use of the Tissue Stress Model as a Paradigm for Developing an Examination and Management Plan for a Patient with Plantar Fasciitis." *Journal of the American Podiatric Medical Association*, 92, no. 9 (2002): 499–506.

Roxas, M. "Plantar Fasciitis: Diagnosis and Therapeutic Considerations." *Alternative Medicine Review*, 10, no. 2 (2005): 83–93.

Ryan, M. B., G. A. Valiant, K. McDonald, and J. E. Taunton. "The Effect of Three Different Levels of Footwear Stability on Pain Outcomes in Women Runners: A Randomised Control Trial." *British Journal of Sports Medicine*, 45, no. 9 (2010): 715–721.

Ryan, M., M. Elashi, R. Newsham-West, and J. Taunton. "Examining Injury Risk and Pain Perception in Runners Using Minimalist Footwear." *British Journal of Sports Medicine*, 48, no. 16 (2014): 1257–1262.

Sabir, N., S. Demirlenk, B. Yagci, N. Karabulut, and S. Cubukcu. "Clinical Utility of Sonography in Diagnosing Plantar Fasciitis." *Journal of Ultrasound in Medicine*, 24, no. 8 (2005): 1041–1048.

Sackett, D. L., W. M. C. Rosenberg, J. A. M. Gray, R. B. Haynes, and W. S. Richardson. "Evidence-Based Medicine: What It Is and What It Isn't." *British Medical Journal*, 312, no. 7023 (1996): 71–72.

Segal, N. A., E. R. Boyer, P. Teran-Yengle, N. A. Glass, H. J. Hillstrom, and H. J. Yack. "Pregnancy Leads to Lasting Changes in Foot Structure." *American Journal of Physical Medicine & Rehabilitation*, 92, no. 3 (2013): 232–240.

Snow, S. W., W. H. O. Bohne, E. DiCarlo, and V. K. Chang. "Anatomy of the Achilles Tendon and Plantar Fascia in Relation to the Calcaneus in Various Age Groups." *Foot & Ankle International*, 16, no. 7 (1995): 418–421.

Snow, D. M., J. Reading, and R. Dalal. "Lateral Plantar Nerve Injury Following Steroid Injection for Plantar Fasciitis." *British Journal of Sports Medicine*, 39, no. e41 (2005): 1–2.

Speed, C. "A Systematic Review of Shockwave Therapies in Soft Tissue Conditions: Focusing on the Evidence." *British Journal of Sports Medicine*, 48 (2014): 1538–1542.

Tatli, Y. Z., and S. Kapasi. "The Real Risks of Steroid Injection for Plantar Fasciitis, with a Review of Conservative Therapies." *Current Reviews in Musculoskeletal Medicine*, 2, no. 1 (2009): 3–9.

Taunton, J. E., M. B. Ryan, D. B. Clement, D. C. McKenzie, D. R. Lloyd-Smith, and B. D. Zumbo, B. D. "A Prospective Study of Running Injuries: The Vancouver Sun Run 'in Training' Clinics." *British Journal of Sports Medicine*, 37, no. 1 (2003): 239–244.

Teyhen, D., and J. Robertson. "Heel Pain." *Journal of Orthopaedic & Sports Physical Therapy*, 41, no. 2 (2011): 51.

Thomas, J. L., J. C. Christensen, S. R. Kravitz, R. W. Mendicino, J. M. Schuberth, J. V. Vanore, … J. Baker. "The Diagnosis and Treatment of Heel Pain: A Clinical Practice Guideline-Revision 2010." *Journal of Foot and Ankle Surgery*, 49, no. 3 (2010): S1–S19.

Tracey, J., S. Allain, A. Dong, R. Josefchak, and J. W. Stewart. Ontario Medical Association. "The Role of the Primary Care Physician in Timely Return to Work." *Ontario Medical Review*, (March 2009): 23–38.

Tsai, W. C., C. C. Hsu, C. P. C. Chen, M. J. L. Chen, T. Y. Yu, and Y. J. Chen. "Plantar Fasciitis Treated with Local Steroid Injection: Comparison between Sonographic and Palpation Guidance." *Journal of Clinical Ultrasound*, 34, no. 1 (2006): 12–16.

Waclawski, E. R., J. Beach, A. Milne, E. Yacyshyn, and D. M. Dryden. "Systematic Review: Plantar Fasciitis and Prolonged Weight Bearing." *Occupational Medicine*, 65, no. 2 (2015): 97–106.

Walther, M., B. Kratschmer, J. Verschl, C. Volkering, S. Altenberger, S. Kriegelstein, and M. Hilgers. Effect of different orthotic concepts as first-line treatment of plantar fasciitis. *Foot and Ankle Surgery*, 19, no. 1 (2013): 103–107.

Wearing, S. C., J. E. Smeathers, S. R. Urry, E. Hennig, and A. P. Hills. "The Pathomechanics of Plantar Fasciitis." Sports Medicine, 36, no. 7 (2006): 585–611.

Wearing, S. C., J. E. Smeathers, B. Yates, P. M. Sullivan, S. R. Urry, and P. Dubois. "Sagittal Movement of the Medial Longitudinal Arch Is Unchanged in Plantar Fasciitis." *Medicine and Science in Sports and Exercise*, 36, no. 10 (2004): 1761–1767.

Werner, R. A., N. Gell, A. Hartigan, N. Wiggerman, and W. M. Keyserling. (2010). "Risk Factors for Plantar Fasciitis Among Assembly Plant Workers." *Physical Medicine & Rehabilitation*, 2, no. 2 (2010): 110–116.

Wheeler, P., K. Boyd, and M. Shipton. "Surgery for Patients with Recalcitrant Plantar Fasciitis: Good Results at Short-, Medium-, and Long-Term Follow-Up." *Orthopaedic Journal of Sports Medicine*, 2, no. 3 (2014): 1–6.

Williams, A. E., A. Martinez-Santos, J. McAdam, and C. J. Nester. "'Trial and Error…,' '…Happy Patients' and '…An Old Toy in the Cupboard': A Qualitative Investigation of Factors That Influence Practitioners in Their Prescription of Foot Orthoses." *Journal of Foot and Ankle Research*, 9, no. 1 (2016): 11–18.

Wong, H. J., and M. Anitescu. "The Role of Health Locus of Control in Evaluating Depression and Other Comorbidities in Patients with Chronic Pain Conditions, a Cross-Sectional Study." *Pain Practice*, (2016): 1–10.

Wrobel, J. S., A. Fleischer, R. T. Crews, B. Jarrett, and B. Najafi. "A Randomized Controlled Trial of Custom Foot Orthoses for the Treatment of Plantar Heel Pain." *Journal of American Podiatric Medical Association*, 105, no. 4 (2015): 281–294.

Young, C. "In the Clinic: Plantar Fasciitis." *Annals of Internal Medicine*, 156, no. 1 (2012): 1–16.

Yucel, I., K. E. Ozturan, Y. Demiraran, E. Degirmenci, and G. Kaynak. "Comparison of High-Dose Extracorporeal Shockwave Therapy and Intralesional Corticosteroid Injection in the Treatment of Plantar Fasciitis." *Journal of the American Podiatric Medical Association*, 100, no. 2 (2010): 105–110.

Yucel, I., B. Yazici, E. Degirmenci, B. Erdogmus, and S. Dogan. "Comparison of Ultrasound-, Palpation-, and Scintigraphy-Guided Steroid Injections in the Treatment of Plantar Fasciitis." *Archives of Orthopaedic and Trauma Surgery*, 129, no. 5 (2009): 695–701.

Yung-Hui, L., and H. Wei-Hsien. "Effects of Shoe Inserts and Heel Height on Foot Pressure, Impact Force, and Perceived Comfort during Walking." *Applied Ergonomics*, 36, no. 3 (2005): 355–362.

ABOUT THE AUTHOR

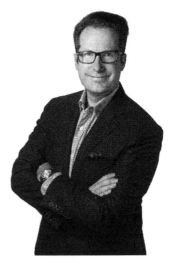

Dr. Colin Dombroski, PhD has managed over six thousand cases of plantar fasciitis since 2002. As Canada's only Canadian-certified pedorthist with a PhD in Health and Rehabilitation Science, Dr. Dombroski runs SoleScience (www.solescience.ca), where he and his team provide custom foot orthoses and pedorthic services. In 2014, *Business London* named him one of the top twenty under forty. An international lecturer and researcher, Dr. Dombroski serves as an adjunct research professor at Western University and acts as a clinical and lab placement instructor in the diploma of pedorthics program. He lives in London, Ontario, with his young family and two Labradors.

Made in the USA
Columbia, SC
06 May 2021

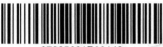